SALLY SEIFFER

the story I tell

how to make the age of disruption work for you

Sally & Sifer

day.

Contents

Preface

No prologue goes unread by me. I love a good backstory. I love broad context to give meaning. Every 'situation' has a backstory. Every human, every living thing, every 'thing' has a story.

Context.

When we are consumed, stuck or spinning, and reacting to life we miss the context – we miss the bigger picture, the broad view. Situations become isolated events that we respond to in often very scripted or routine ways. People become the role they are assigned by the perceiver, or perceivers. People become the role they assign themselves, consciously or unconsciously, as the receiver. The roles have rules as to how we act and respond. We become these robots, these vessels of predictable routine and behavior.

This is not living. This is not alive.

In Part one, I share my early experience working as a school mental health provider. I felt powerless in response to student death by suicide and school violence. I share my aha moment that came at the end of a school year which included two suicide deaths. After receiving the news the second time, I paced my kitchen floor and questioned the silence, 'what do we do?' The answer I received was, 'Life. Sell life.'

The story goes on to tell that I realized I was not alive. I was not living. I had been experiencing a cycle of depression that would come and go every two weeks, and it had gone on for over a decade. I realized that if I could figure out the skills to get my own life back, then I would know the skills to teach others. The skills that worked. The skills that contributed toward life and sustainable growth. Lasting.

In Part two, Keeley tells a story of love, without conditions attached to the love. Great love. Keeley is a dog. My dog. The dog I received. The lessons she taught me are easy to see now that she has been dead for almost seven years. The story of Keeley represents something more. Something bigger. We all certainly must have Keeleys around us all the time, everywhere. 'Keeley' exists. Love exists. We just choose to open up to it.

Love transmits. It has to be received. To turn away from love and possibility is suffering.

In Part three, I share some fundamental skills, tools, and strategies that created shifts in my thinking, and transformed my experience of ordinary life. Self-awareness helped me recognize my limiting thoughts. When I changed my thinking, I changed the story. I created my own script. I chose the filter. The new story created new feelings. I felt good. And I knew why. I knew how to create it and sustain it. It felt extraordinary to be so empowered.

I have been out of the depression cycle for over three years. I publish a weekly blog, *STuFfeD: self-care 101*. The tagline is 'ordinary day...extraordinary way'. My definition of self-care is to care about yourself enough to notice your thoughts. What story do they tell? Limiting stories lead to limiting outcomes. Expansive thoughts, rooted in possibility, lead to expansive feelings and results. Results that are able to sustain themselves. Results that continue to grow, to expand. Evolve.

The practice of self-awareness, or mindfulness, allows one to disrupt stories that don't edify and contribute toward life-giving outcomes. *Personal Growth* content can be reduced to one primary stance: tell your own story.

I

why.

As a human who feels the world much better than she can articulate it, it's important for me to share the 'why'. The outcomes in school need to change. And they will. I wish for a world where students are fully engaged in their day – in all aspects of day. Ordinary day...extraordinary way. Now THIS is me.

skills.

As I continually aspire to find a sequence to my content, I return to a moment in a school office years back. It was an interesting time of change in the school district I was working in – there had been a massive budget mistake that froze salaries at about the same time the housing recession hit. For a variety of reasons, 'fear' was a theme. Fear of losing your job due to budget cuts, fear of not addressing the needs of a student's IEP and being the one responsible for the ensuing litigation, fear of being responsible for not taking the necessary steps to address a student's health and wellbeing that resulted in their death by suicide, fear of being responsible for a school shooting – not addressing the signs.

Fear.

So all that was going on, and I was a brand new school social worker. As a school social worker, I feel as if I can speak on behalf of most whom work in Denver and the greater Denver area – we are not prepared for the role of a school mental health provider as it relates specifically to IDEA (special education law). Because I had little to no understanding of what it meant to be a special service provider on an IEP, I stuck to what I did know – teaching social and emotional curriculum, and 'meeting kids where they were at'.

My office was conveniently located in the main office where guidance counseling lived – so there was no shortage of students that showed up wanting to talk to a busy school counselor. Since I really had no set schedule (I didn't get the whole SPED thing) I was available for students. To move this story along - I got really good at doing suicide assessments. To be really good at suicide assessments includes a few main things:

1. Willing to sit with the student and be present, to listen with the intent to hear.
2. Willing to ask direct questions and be okay with the answer.
3. Able to fill out the suicide risk assessment and follow the process that is laid out for you.
4. Make a phone call home to a 'parent'.
5. Transfer the student to the hospital when necessary.

Essentially you could say the same thing about threat/risk assessments. The processes are great.

But then what?

Obviously there is more to effective suicide assessment and intervention - and there are wonderful trainings and programs to support the issue and the processes.

The point in stating the above is that there was a process. Processes are great in the work environment - and probably in lots of other environments as well.

Processes give boundaries, lay a worn path, and allow for some routine and/or expectation. However, as it relates to suicidal ideation...there is more going on, clearly. Being really good at the 1-5 list is helpful, and people at work will like someone who is competent at addressing and moving toward the uncomfortable experience of students in this emotional state - but what is the change agent? What can be done to alleviate or lessen the outcome? When the student returns to school, we fill out a reentry form and create a safety plan. But what are the skills to teach in moving forward toward effective growth and sustainable outcomes?

Back to the 'moment' in the school office. I have this mental picture of myself. I could close the door and shut the blinds. Now and again I would do that. Sometimes I just needed a break. Other times I sat and cried because I didn't know how to help. One moment stuck with me, and I remember so vividly asking out loud to the emptiness of the space - 'what are the skills?'

I knew that I had gotten to a point where I had some validity in my competencies to do a job - maybe not the job SPED required - (the one I am quite familiar with now at the elementary level), but I was good at crisis, good at the extra - connecting and teaching social and emotional curriculum in the classroom setting, addressing the needs of students with undesirable behavior or lagging skills in managing emotions at school, being part of problem solving and expulsion programs, etc.

What happened in that office was a very raw and honest recognition that what I was doing was okay - but it wasn't getting to the core. I wasn't familiar with the effective skills (and affective) that got different results - that helped those hurting to manage the *Big Feelings*. What. Were. The. Skills.???????

I have always seen a bigger picture. I have always laughed at the context of humor more than maybe just the joke. I could see the greater need for teaching skills to disrupt the end results. I did not know what the skills were. I was convinced that I just happened to miss it - I didn't pay attention when I was taught the skills, or I didn't take 'the class' where the magical skills were taught.

So this is where I begin.

"What are the skills?" she asks herself over and over again. What are the skills that disrupt the undesirable outcomes?

life.

When the phone rings at a certain time in the morning, before you have left for work, and the person calling is an administrator at the school you work at - it is usually not good. I'm pretty sure I had dreaded this particular phone call ever since I became a school social worker. And I'm not sure if it was for the right reasons.

Maybe at first it was just that I felt ill-equipped to handle something with the magnitude that crisis brings. I know at some point my concern became one of fear - fear that I was going to be responsible for the crisis...the student death by suicide, or a violent act that could have been prevented had I done my job right.

The phone call I dreaded was received early in the school year - the last school year I worked full time in a high school. A ninth grade student had completed suicide. Sadly, the first reaction I had was relief - relief that it wasn't a student I had been working with. I suppose the first reaction was fear - 'oh shit'. And then came the relief. Not because it would be 'sad' because I had a relationship with the student, nope. It was because I would feel responsible for the student's death.

I like to think the truth is that I experienced a range of feelings. I know, after receiving the call and processing that initial reaction of fear, my thoughts went straight to the family experience. What was it like to find her, to tell her siblings, and all the 'next steps' I could conceive of. This 'empathy' experience hits hard and lasts long - the feeling experience of this 'compassion' thing that most of us in the mental health field have in abundance - the sensory experience that feels as if it is happening to you...feeling all the feelings.

I would be lying if I shared anything other than my initial reaction - oh shit, am I responsible? 'Am I going to get in trouble?' It's silly, right? And so very rooted in a thinking pattern that can begin so young - am I going to get in trouble? Did I do something wrong?

It's curious why that is. Why is it that in a school environment the first reaction is so closely linked to the whole CYA (cover-your-ass) mindset. Fear. I knew that this was the disconnect. I'm not sure if I started teasing this out prior to the student death or after. It really doesn't matter. I knew the processes put in place were helpful. Yet, there is still the something else - the something more. Something was off. If we could 'chip away' at the offness when it comes to addressing these issues, maybe we could get closer to unmasking the pathway to healthy and sustainable outcomes.

I got two phone calls during this particular school year. The next one came at the end of the year and the student was on life support. I got off the phone and I remember pacing my kitchen floor.

I wanted different outcomes. I wanted to figure out how to get different results. Something was off and the focus of intervention needed to match that - whatever 'that' was. The human piece.

All of a sudden I projected audibly in the kitchen with arms in the air - life! This is the answer. If death is the focus of the 'problem' then life is the solution. We 'sell' life! That's the solution. This epiphany at some point led me back to me. Was I alive? If I was going to begin to sell this idea of life to teenagers...what was I going to sell? Was I living a life of vitality and active, healthy engagement in balanced pursuits that were as enjoyable as they were meaningful and uplifting? Oh HELL no...I was not alive.

At some point, I realized that if I could figure out how to 'live' and what the 'skills' were to return this 'life' back to me, THEN I would understand what these magical skills were that led to the healthy and sustainable GROWTH outcomes that made sense – the something more. The human piece.

share.

I gave away the gist of this chapter in the previous chapter. My 'lightbulb is on' - aha moment came when I realized that if the 'problem' is death and the desire to die, then the answer is life and the desire to live.

Death. Dying. And the desire to die. Dead.

Life. Living. And the desire to live. Alive.

I'm not sure of the exact timing the depth of the insight really hit me. The next level realization came when I visualized myself facilitating the risk assessments. The person on the other side (me) was not alive. Ironically, I could see the life in the student that was sitting across from me. More specifically, I could feel it.

When I looked at them in these assessments, I would feel what I have named 'the gush'. An expansive, open feeling, a knowing...what I would call love. Love without conditions put on it. I always assumed it was what their parents must feel when they looked at them - until the number of kids I spent time with included kids who did not have the 'parent' present...which made the whole gush somewhat of a mystery - but it felt good, so it didn't really matter what its orientation was. It felt right. It felt very much alive. It felt like what I would call 'truth'. I wanted the student to feel what I felt. I wanted to know how to transfer this 'knowing' that they were okay. If they could feel what I felt, they too would know they're okay.

As easily as I could sense this 'love' during the time I spent with the students, particularly during these 1:1 meetings, I couldn't find this feeling toward myself. The thought of thinking or caring about myself this way was disconnected. It seemed unrecognizable, but also unreasonable. I needed to suffer. I needed to be in opposition to myself – to hold my own self accountable for my mistakes and shortcomings. I needed to be critical and judgmental of myself because that is somehow justified as morally sound and 'right'. I was depressed. I was unhappy. I was not alive.

I realized that if I really desired to uncover the skills that led to authentic and lasting outcomes that would change the results of student death by suicide and school violence, then I had an opportunity to uncover, apply, and practice the skills on me. If I could discover the skills, tools, and strategies that returned life to me, then it would be easy to share them with others. Now it was about finding the skills.

The students were being prescribed Dialectical Behavior Therapy (DBT) when they were seen at the emergency room for self harm, or when they were released after being hospitalized. DBT appeared to be a series of weekly group sessions held at the hospital. At the time, the hospital was miles away from the high school I was located. Let's just say that the students were not attending the sessions with any sort of fidelity. I figured this DBT could be a starting point. What was DBT? What were the skills?

DBT

Here we are on the last piece of the 'why'. Why blog. Why throw up content on a Facebook Page and a YouTube channel. Why host a store on Teacher Pay Teacher. Why online courses. Why?

It all began with a desire for effective outcomes. What were the skills that resulted in new ways of experiencing *Big Feelings*. *Big Feelings* is a term I began using as my 'job' transitioned to elementary school. I use the term *Big Feelings* to describe the feelings that show up uninvited, and are in no hurry to leave. It began with the desire to teach skills that got sustainable results, and I realized that life was the answer. I was doing so many suicide assessments, and the irony was that I was not alive myself. I was not present. Happy. Satisfied. *Big Feelings* were in charge of me, and had been for a long time. If I could figure out the skills, apply them to my own situation, and get lasting results – then I had the answer. I would know what skills work, and transfer the teachings to the students.

Here is the rest of the story.

Once I seemed to have the strategy figured out, I decided to start with Dialectical Behavior Therapy (DBT). The skills I was looking for must exist inside DBT – this seemed to be what the students were being 'prescribed' when they were seen medically for self harm and suicidal behaviors.

If I am recalling correctly, I googled 'DBT' in my office, in an urgent state of mind ('this must happen now!') and I wrote down the skills. These would be the skills I focus on. I still may have the little piece of ripped off notebook paper that I scribbled the skills on. Honestly, I don't remember the exact language of the skill sets that make up DBT because my story resonates with the one skill that was completely unknown to me at the time - mindfulness.

I jotted down the 4 skills, and decided to focus on the skills that made sense (skills such as anxiety reduction, conflict resolution, social skill building... skills like that).

That summer was a breaking point for crazy. I hated my job. I hated where I lived. I hated the boy I had been in a relationship with for about a year and a half. I say I hated those things - I hated me. I hated my patterns. I hated that I couldn't get it together. I hated that I had a longing for something more and I had no clue what it was. I moved out of my place, and put my belongings in storage. Sent the boy a text to say I needed a break (yes I texted as a preemptive move because I was so emotional). That was that. I didn't quit my job - I wanted to (that lasted one more school year). I stayed in a coworker's family cabin in Breckenridge with my dog for all of June and July.

When I drove up the mountain and was driving into town, I stopped at the library. The summer was going to be meaningful. I was going to change. At the library, they had books for sale. *Mindfulness.* Wait...what? That word. *Mindfulness.* Of course I bought the book. To be honest, the book was really uneventful that summer. It was too simple. The language was written for a first grader. A Vietnemese monk wrote the book and it was translated into English. I figured something must have been lost in translation.

Thich Nhat Hanh.

Mindfulness.

Simple.

The practice changed my life. I wish I could tell you it all happened that summer. I was certain that it did. That I was forever changed, and moving forward would be done in a perpetual state of bliss. I did change. Oh did I change. I am so appreciative that I had that summer to get away and experience the time in the backdrop of so much beauty.

The turning of 40 and the Breckenridge summer is the timestamp I use to suggest the significance of my turning point. Anyone that has life changing experiences (I think) can look back and realize that it wasn't just the event, situation, or circumstance. Sure, there was something that finally got your attention. It's all of it. All the moving parts and pieces – and it continues to move. The desire for something more, and the experience that finally brings you back to you.

I get it. My personal 'big events' don't seem too tragic or too traumatic. And at this point, I have learned how to tell a different story. The story I want to tell. A story that is grounded in possibility. So unless I need to share something in a way that contributes to the point I'm trying to make – I'm not going to focus on the suffering. Yes, I did move toward the suffering. Yes, I made peace with the suffering. The healing is in the flow of possibility. To shift, or to pivot away, from what you don't want into the feeling state of what you do want.

And again, anyone who has had to meet suffering by choice or by force, I think they will tell you that when it gets to that point – the desired outcome is no longer something that is tangible. It's not something that can be quantified, not something that can be boxed up and shipped. It's a feeling. In my case, nothing else mattered outside of the inside feeling of freedom.

At the low point, I really believed that I could handle ANYTHING if I could just feel free inside. If I was free inside, I could manage anything external.

So that's the why. That's the story behind my project.

Day.

Simple and transferable skills, tools, and strategies to grow wellbeing.

Ordinary day...extraordinary way.

Now THIS is me.

II

love.

the something more.

"Now, scholars can be very useful and necessary, in their own dull and amusing way. They provide a lot of information. It's just that there is Something More, and that Something More is what life is really all about."

the tao of pooh

keeley.

Michellie.

Pronounced Muh-kee-lee.

Keeley for short.

Keeley was my first conscious understanding of what pure, whole, honest love must feel like.

I was living in Hemet, California. When asked about Hemet, I would refer to it as the poor man's Palm Springs. It was a relatively small (but not small) and growing town west of the San Jacinto mountain range - the other side of Palm Springs. I had just bought a home. It was in the midst of the southern California housing boom. My co worker friend and I went to look at some new builds during lunch. I found a one story, three bedroom that was being constructed. I walked into the trailer, and said I wanted it. I wrote them a $100 check for a home I later received $77,000.00 that paid for graduate school tuition, just over two years later (and that was after I had refinanced - original price $172,000, sold $310,000...it was a good time to buy a home in S. Cali).

The small housing development was on a river bed. The river bed, which was mostly dry, was observable from an easily navigated 'cliff' behind my across-the-street neighbor's backyard. It was a massive expanse of open land - no buildings or civilization in sight, just the front range terrain of the San

Jacintos. I was a runner at the time, and the expanse of land was drool worthy. An organic path system had been formed. You could see natural pathways from the lookout on the cliff, they followed the dry river bed. The land was an Indian reservation. The Soboba Indian Reservation had its share of 'tales' that I had heard about - what happens on the land stays on the land, sort of tales. The only thing the 'tales' did for my naive 31 year old self was suggest that I needed a partner to navigate the land with.

I was playing Bunco with a group of teachers and their 'others' from my best friend's elementary school. Bunco. Teachers. Yep. It was actually a lot of fun. On one Bunco night, there was mention of a pregnant dog. A pregnant purebred boxer who stayed in a cage outside - a large cage that was part of a gorgeous fenced in pool and outdoor living space. The home was further away from where I lived, but it was built on a massive expanse of land that also spawned from the San Jacintos. All this land was being developed, the housing boom was in full force, a lot of wild was being disrupted. The pure bred boxer got knocked up. The hunch was something 'wild' had shown up in the night.

And then came Keeley.

I visited the puppies shortly after they were born. There were two distinct types - half were big and white with fluffy fur, and the other half were smaller, tan with white spots - not so fluffy. I chose one of the 'not so fluffies' with a white necklace marking around its neck. The dog owners had a little boy. I told the little boy which one I wanted. He told me later that he put Keeley in his bed at night. I picked up Keeley at 5 weeks old. Clueless. The puppy still slept mostly, and moved seldom. I had nothing - no blanket, nothing. I laid it on the passenger seat. It didn't move.

I had no intention of ever writing this story. I suppose I also had no intention of ever not writing this story. It is a story that lives inside of me. It feels emotional to share as I type the words, but not because it's sad. Keeley isn't alive, and hasn't been for some time. The emotion dwelling up, as the memories surface, is the emotion of love. The gush x 100.

The gush is the inside, felt experience of what I call love. Expansive, open, light, free. A feeling unattached to conditions or outcomes. It exists. It shows up. It just is. We 'get' to feel it.

I became quite familiar with the gush when I received Keeley. I didn't have a name for it, but something was happening on the inside of me that was strong. It was stronger, and got my attention, more than anything else I had experienced up to this time. I realized at some point that what I was feeling must be the inner experience of pure love. There was no transaction between Keeley and I. Keeley existed. The feeling wasn't synthetic, something I could make more or less of necessarily. I couldn't hug her enough, give kisses enough, or tell her enough. I had to just have the feeling. I 'got' to just have the feeling. I could 'do' nothing but surrender to the feeling. Allow the feeling. The feeling was present when I was present with it.

By comparison, I think with other humans, or even with other living systems, there is this actionable quality associated with 'love'. Little did I know at the time, I was entering into a rough ten year period. I say 'rough' because I am exposed to other people's 'rough' on a daily, and in hindsight, my 'rough' doesn't seem to compare. But. Feelings are feelings. And dark, empty, obsessive, controlling, hateful energy in motion (emotion) sucks no matter what the story attached reads like. As I went through the next ten years, I ironically - but obviously, so not ironically - got to do it with Keeley. Easy to see...now.

It's funny with dogs, we think we are in charge. We think our pet is so fortunate to have us. So easy to recognize now that love was ever present during my (what felt like) endless process of undoing, and exposing, the limiting, destructive stories that I was telling...about me.

wild.

I love this word.

To be wild is to be free. To not be held captive to other's ideas, expectations, rules. Like all words, 'wild' holds a vibration. An energy. A current. To some, the word wild might suggest a different interpretation that feels uncomfortable, out of control. A wild fire. 'The kids are acting wild' - unable to be contained. 'The crowd went wild.'

I became curious about the word 'wild' the summer after I had my first official teaching year at Cary-Grove high school in Cary, Illinois. I had the wonderful opportunity to grow up in Cary, and attend Cary-Grove high school. When I was hired to teach at the high school, there were still a number of teachers who had taught me as a student. One of the teachers, Francey Zender, was wild. Francey lived by herself in an apartment just outside of Cary. Francey taught Humanities 1 & 2 at CGHS. Francey's wisdom and expansive thinking was lost on me as a high school student, and I can't say I was completely absorbed as a twenty-something-first-year-teacher to what Francey had to offer. Francey loved me. My guess is that she picked up on my energy - my potential. I like to think I do the same with students that show up in my experience - you feel their truth. Words and actions become largely irrelevant...you pick up on a feeling, a spirit. Teacher becoming the space holder of love and possibility.

So when Francey, whom had received a reputation amongst students in my generation to be one of the 'it' teachers (I hadn't picked up on the why - I think she was the Dead Poet Society version to CGHS in the 80's for sure...again, lost on me), when she shared with me a flyer on a 6-credit hour English course offering out of Northern Illinois University, that was to be held in the Tarryall mountain range located in Colorado, I was certain that this would grow me and my enlightenment. Let's just say that at the time I wasn't too sure what enlightenment even meant.

Francey never shared her age. I tried to peek at her driver's license when we rented our fly fishing equipment. I think I figured it to be 77. Badass.

The course included six reads to be completed prior to the 3-week experience taking place in the mountains. The books would be discussed at campfire throughout the trip.

As you may assume, the books were stories about the experience of the wild. I can only remember two - Annapurna and Into the Wild. They might have been the only two I read, although I like to think at the ripe old age of 26 I had matured enough to read all six as per course requirements. Whatever.

The 3-week Colorado trip was to allow for the experience of what the stories from the books shared. Let's be honest, there were two English professors at NIU, one had a lifetime friend who owned a base camp in the Tarryalls', both professors passionate about the outdoors. They created the course - a paid adventure.

We took two backpack excursions, one for three sleeps, and the other for five. I had never slept in a tent. We even did a solo sleep sans tent. This wasn't the first time I jumped in the deep end before learning how to swim. I still have the tendency. Rock climbing, and car camp trips, to explore some lesser popularized areas of Colorado were driven to and experienced. I bouldered, I climbed, I fly-fished (hated it). I mountain-biked. I even ended up in a care clinic to have the scree washed out of my left ass after I had endo'd on a mountain bike ride and, when landed on my feet, only had more adrenaline that proved to be too much, as I next hit a rock and lost control - tossed off the bike to slide down a portion of the path. The scree embedded up my left thigh into my butt cheek (had I been wearing spandex this would not have been an issue). I kind of felt cool - but not when it was scrubbed out - nor did I feel cool when the healing process was juicy and smelled, and would continue to rip open and bleed every time I got up out of the car on the road trip back to Illinois. The medic on duty in Woodland Park had held my leg down like a chicken wing, and scrubbed me out like the bottom of a baking dish that hadn't soaked long enough. All this happened while I scream-laughed at a volume 15 (scale to 10) - the Bill Clinton impeachment trial taking place in the background... 'I did not have sexual relations...'

I'm getting a little carried away in these stories that took place well over a decade ago - a decade? 26? um...over two decades... all because of this present time topic, *love,* and my love teacher - Michellie (Keeley). Keeley was not in existence yet. I wouldn't move back to California the second time for another four years. The point of the summer mountain English class trip is to talk about 'wild'. It was at a campfire conversation that I was exposed to new thinking: what does wild mean to you?

Keeley. Wild. Untamed.

Love.

impermanence.

I think most dog owners can look back at their dog's life and point to lessons learned. In my case, the broad lesson, or theme, was the conscious experience of what love without conditions feels like. Now I recognize that love without conditions just 'is'. It is an energy that exists. We can call it wellbeing, infinite intelligence, spirit, flow, etc. It exists within laws that govern that energy. The awareness and understanding of impermanence was second to the lesson of unconditional love. Impermanence being the lesson that stubbornly revealed energy as dynamic, flowing, ever-changing...form and formless.

In the school setting, working with elementary age, there is a stage of development where the students' recognize impermanence. This can be a difficult shift for children. Any 'shift' of a belief allows for change. Change and trauma go hand in hand in my opinion. My generalized definition of trauma is that it has a range, and is experienced on different levels by most people. Trauma is a life event, circumstance, or situation that was unexpected, and changed one's experience of what was assumed to be 'normal'. The result of trauma is some level of emotional dysregulation, and (what seems to be) a lack of control, to varying degrees, over the dysregulation.

Impermanence is the recognition that life energy is dynamic, ever-changing. Things are not meant to be one way and stay. Can you see how this one contrary belief about permanence, and the mindset we create around it, could unintentionally lead toward outcomes (observable behavior and the results that show up) that resonate with one's need to control outcomes that, by nature and the laws that guide it, cannot be controlled?

Keeley was maybe six years old when I realized this wasn't a forever thing, she and I. I was going out of town, and a nearby veterinary clinic had a kennel. For Keeley to stay at the kennel, she had to have a wellness examination. I think this is how the story goes. She had a 'tooth thing'. The vet lifted up her gum, and her back tooth was covered up by the gum - swollen, red. They were going to pull the tooth, and until they did it was uncertain what the significance of the 'tooth thing' was - the 'c' word was mentioned. I went on the trip wondering for the first time, what if this was all the time I would have with Keeley?

There was no significance to the 'tooth thing', I went on to forget about being present and attuned, and Keeley went on to get really overweight and began to lose chunks of fur on her back. If impermanence is the chapter theme, then this segment theme is denial.

There was nothing I loved more than Keeley. How was it that she gained 20 lbs (on a dog body) and literally had at least four, maybe six, relatively large chunks of fur no longer attached to her, resulting in large, black, grinch-skin-like open patches. The weight and the skin patches were present for months before finally one night in bed, petting her, with huge chunks of fur coming out in my hand, I realized there was a problem.

Back to the vet. The vet had told me at the initial tooth thing, that Keeley needed to lose weight. Denied. Now the vet had my attention, and I realized that she needed to lose weight. How do I help her lose weight? I asked. BY NOT FEEDING HER MORE THAN WHAT WAS APPROPRIATE FOR HER SIZE. Ohhhh...the table scraps, the endless treats given out of guilt for being gone all day? Wait, I am the one responsible for the weight? Weight was only one thing. She also had a thyroid problem which she would begin to take medication daily, lasting the rest of her life.

You may think I'd have 'woken up' and began to 'pay attention' a bit more. The next incident came on a walk. I noticed that she had huge growth of her anal glands. When did this happen? She looked like a boy dog from behind.

The last and most significant event happened, and finally got my attention. Literally, got my attention. I was now awake. It was after the Breckenridge summer. October.

I was busy. When Keeley was having these 'situations' occur, I could have noticed ahead of time had I been 'attuned' to her and 'present'. I was working two jobs. I worked full-time at a high school, and then worked part-time at an alternative high school setting that started at 3:15pm. I loved working at the alternative school setting. It fit because the students I spent time with at the day school were transferring to the evening school to gain credits to graduate. Still. Too much. And my focus was totally skewed. I was miserable - but I had yet to realize that I was the one who could change it.

I had the big Breckenridge summer awakening, and moved into my cool duplex off 6th avenue in Denver. I was working the two jobs, so my paycheck 'looked' good - it looked like what I should have been making in one job (I mentioned that pay had been frozen years prior and continued to stay the same). I was 'thin' - I knew this because all my clothes fit after a summer of Crossfit, running, swimming, hiking and my version of a paleo-ish diet that was popular with Crossfit. Great. I was enlightened, and creating my perfect life. No more *Big Feelings*. Riiiight.

Fall Break. Busy. Didn't buy Keeley dog food. In the week leading up to break, I switched dog food on Keeley three times. She had started doing the deep, tummy, pre-throw up thing. Denial. Not a good time to get sick Keeley. You're okay.

I dropped Keeley off at a different kennel situation that was in a big warehouse close to the airport. She had been there before. The owners were hardcore dog people.

I left for the airport. I landed in Florida. Parents picked me up, and we stopped at a restaurant in Fort Myers. Ah. Now it was time to relax. Checked my phone. The kennel called. Keeley's stomach had twisted due to the discomfort and her 'throwing up' thing – all the gas created this space for her tummy to bounce around and then twist, cutting off the flow of oxygen. The dog people were aware of the twisted tummy, as it happens to dogs of a certain size. Keeley was now at the emergency vet, and her 'numbers' were all over the place. The vet I spoke with told me that 'putting her down' was a reasonable option.

So now I was present. I loved Keeley. It was not something I could explain. I felt it. Keeley was my set point. Keeley existed. I had Keeley to return to when the other things were feeling out of my control. I wanted to say goodbye to Keeley. I remember being in the bedroom at my parents – sobbing. I couldn't see in my mind's eye the markings on her body. I wondered how I could love something so much, but be so unaware of what she actually looked like. I had this thought that if Keeley could live through this then I was going to know her markings. I was going to be present and attuned, and appreciate this dog.

By now, I have probably lost you if you aren't a dog person. Drama. If you are a dog person, you most likely get the love thing. If you are human, on some level I'm guessing the attunement and presence resonates. How is it that these things we love are also things that we...wait for it...might...take for granted (?)

I spoke with the vet on duty through the night – she had just gotten on shift when we originally spoke. She was going to call me if it was imminent to put Keeley down – obviously I didn't want Keeley to suffer just so I could get my ass back to Denver to say goodbye. Gawd I wanted to see her, touch her, hold her, whisper to her what she meant to me and how thankful I was to have her as my dog.

I got the first flight back the next morning. Funny (now) story. The flight I booked was going out of Tampa. My parents had picked me up in Ft Myers the evening before. They live in between the two airports, about thirty minutes closer to Ft Myers. On the way to the airport that morning I was obviously upset and distracted. I finally noticed the sign on the road said something about Ft Myers airport. "Dad. Are we going to Tampa?" "No, Sal." It was too late to turn around so we went to Ft Myers and I spoke to the ticket agent who got me a ticket out of Ft Lauderdale, across the state. I made the flight within, not kidding, a minute before they shut the door. Headed to Dallas and then home to Keeley.

When I finally got to the vet, prepared for the worst but also kind of knowing that she wasn't done yet. Keeley greeted me as Keeley. Keeley was a nervous dog – (now I interpret the entire experience as all the energy Keeley took on of mine that was totally messed up). Keeley had gone to the kennel, and was then taken to the emergency vet. That's a lot of transition for any dog, especially a nervous dog. The original vet I had spoken with had just returned back on shift. She looked at me and said 'hm. She hasn't been like this since I have seen her.' SO YOU WERE GOING TO PUT HER DOWN!!! – that's another story.

Keeley came home with me. We got her stomach stapled later that week. There were two sleepless nights that I stayed up with her. I was present. I massaged her back gently while she cried like dogs cry when they are hurting. I was present. I allowed the space of love to be what it was and have the experience by choice. Michellie's markings continue to be etched into my memory.

Keeley lived two more years. We continued to run in the mornings up until the Friday before she died (on a Tuesday). She took a daily thyroid pill and now another pill for gas, and was put on a special food that I purchased at the vet.

I did not hesitate to use credit to pay for all things Keeley. I also didn't hesitate to use credit to pay for all things mindfulness. I was determined to end the bullshit *Big Feelings* and teach others how to do it. Next phase: working 3 FTE jobs and a 1.5 workload (yep – paycheck was looking fabulous). And then

I didn't get the full time job I anticipated. I had all this debt and now a job contract for .7…$^{2}/_{3}$'s of a full time contract. This too is another story. A story titled: Bankrupt.

guide.

Over the ten years that I 'got' to have Keeley, I can look back and see the guide that she was. Keeley was an external reference point to what I couldn't yet experience on my own...my set point, my equilibrium.

As discussed and confirmed: I loved Keeley. In the midst of what I would call my suffering, which included me taking on other's energy and not knowing how or what to do with it and, as a result, continuing to feed this powerless state, Keeley held the space of love. The space that exists, the space of wellbeing, of balance, not too much, not too little, enough.

To receive the love, I only needed to be open to it. When you are the dog owner (or the parent, the teacher, the person in the perceived role of power) you assume you are the one in charge, the one that others rely on and need in order to function, to exist. I suppose there is evidence to support this.

When I would get stuck or consumed, I would think of Keeley and feel relief in my body. Love. She existed. I got to go home to Keeley. I got to cuddle with Keeley. Intentionally creating the audible sound of Keeley's breath in my imagination became a skill I used often to slow down when I first began to practice mindfulness.

The interesting thing about dogs, and this experience of love, was that the dog holds this space and all the human can do is allow it. One cannot consume the dog. The dog has these natural boundaries that 'force' you to just accept the feeling, to allow the feeling. This experience is available often in nature when we allow it, when we open up to it. The awe of existence.

Why would someone EVER do something unkind and dismissive of that which they genuinely felt such a pure love for?

Insert judgment.

Insert comparison.

Insert criticism.

Judgement, comparison, and criticism is a double edged sword. An assumption that there is ultimately a right and a wrong. If you have read the story up to this point, you can reference back to the wild section. Keeley and I were wild together in the dry riverbed of the Soboba Indian reservation. Keeley was free - gawd was she ever free, and I desired to be free. What a match. In the riverbed, the unspoken rule was that there were no rules. Everyone who entered did so on their own volition - there were no laws or governing bodies. It was just a huge expansive space of unknown, in Keeley and my case.

And then we moved to Denver.

One of my first desires when I moved to Denver was to find the 'space' to run and be free. I assumed the people in Denver appreciated space and freedom as much as I did - it was the Rocky mountains. The biggest and best dry riverbed EVER!

I did not like to have Keeley on a leash. It seemed totally reasonable, and totally Denver, to me. Let's just say that Denver and Colorado are two different mindsets. For the sake of telling a story, I am creating broad themes that connect to bigger ideas - but I was a nieve, inexperienced, and largely clueless dog owner. I was definitely the owner that assumed all other humans loved and appreciated Keeley as much as I did – how could they not, right? Lesson learned.

I do.not.even. know where and what to tell and share here – there are so many instances. There was the woman at the dog park who told me that my dog was a pit bull and that pit bulls were 'put down' in Denver. It was the law. There were the dog fights...the forever presence of the potential dog fight that I eventually clued into and attempted to steer away from. I just wanted to run free and wanted Keeley to run free. I assumed that dogs had a way that they figure their shit out. Keeley was WILD. I was wild. Together we were a disaster in the open space where laws and rules were to be followed.

The Cherry Creek reservoir open space dog park eventually beat me into submission to the point where I assumed that no other human liked Keeley, that they were all scared of her, and they all judged me to be a lacking, unskilled dog owner that really should not have a dog. So now we go from totally untamed to tame, with no space in the middle.

The projection of what I was going through in my inside world, to my outside world at the time, is becoming even more clear. Keeley's external experience was a reflection of my inner experience that was not available, or I was not available to see it yet. I was in grad school. Holy hell of two years. All previous beliefs – religious and political, dominant views, etc – all completely disrupted – tossed up and spinning wildy in the wind to eventually settle, but not for what seemed an eternity. There was something about grad school from the first seat I took in class. I knew I was there to receive and not share.

There was the time Keeley jumped out of the back car window, the time Keeley took off after something and we lost each other – several walkers had seen a dog howling in the parking lot.. 'I'm coming Keeley!', the multiple times she went after the horses – there were stables connected to the open space park and on the weekends there were family trail rides THROUGH the dog park – (Keeley was not the only one disrupting that situation), there was the time she nipped the butt of the man in the service uniform, the puncture wound to my friend's dog when we arrived after a long trip in the car. The road trips. Many road trips with Keeley.

Keeley and I finally gave up on the open space dog park (much to other's appreciation) and began running on streets using an extended leash really early in the morning. Keeley and I ran most early mornings of most of her life. We also went on crazy long walks quite often on the weekends. I was addicted to movement and exercise, and I felt guilty for not being home so much during the week. So the win-win was running together in the early morning, and then the afternoon early evening walk was bonus.

There had always been moments to capture the love. The space of the dog park held the possibility of freedom, and the moments of bliss. Aside from the mine traps of dog fights and horse chases, there was another riverbed that was often flowing. I had at least a 4 mile open run in the reservoir, with about 2 miles running along the river (maybe 20 feet wide and 3 feet at the deepest, unless there was a lot of rain or snow to really get it moving). I would run on the trail, and Keeley would run through the water. There were pockets of water that were insane for dogs - I called it Doggie Disneyland. I found the 'ponds' that were off the main path. One had a bench. Not sure why not many people and dogs landed there. It might have been that we were there (?) After the run - sometimes I ran it twice, I would sit and Keeley would be in the water. There was plenty of bliss when I was available to it. Oh the space. The sky. The dirt path. The runs that felt so effortless at times. The times it felt like all the suffering was a mistake, and now it would be okay. Not true at the time - my peace was still a ways from being something I knew how to sustain - but it felt so good, I would think to myself in these moments, it had to be like this.

Anxiety had never really been my thing. Depression was it. Depression and anxiety often seem to show up together with the students I have worked with over the years. I had a panic attack, or what I would call a panic attack, one time at the dog park that made me forever empathetic to the students, or to adults, that speak of anxiety. I was in the space of the park. The setting was cued. There was wide open space, I was running, Keeley was behaving. Something just attacked me on the inside. I couldn't escape. All this freedom, space, movement outside and something inside was on attack – I couldn't run fast enough. I couldn't do anything. It had a grip. I think I cried and just kept running, eventually to the car. I'm not sure what happened next. I was years from meditating and having any true skills, other than medication, to help me. I ran. I no longer journaled. I watched Sex and the City. I called my parents and complained which only made it worse. They got upset, and my dad would try to fix it by asking if quitting (grad school) was an option. Not sure about the panic attack – it must have just run its course.

So that's a lot of wild and untamed. When we moved back to the city after the Breckenridge summer, Keeley and I walked and ran in a really nice neighborhood, probably the nicest neighborhood in Denver – Country Club they call it. We steered clear of all other dogs. Moving to the other side of the street way ahead of possible meetings. Avoid.

I was allowing other people the power. Partly, I did need to be a responsible pet owner. The broader piece was my fucked up belief where I continually assumed I was doing something wrong. Never good enough. Never enough. Keeley was not at fault. I didn't teach Keeley. I was the fuck up.

the end.

The last few weeks of Keeley's life had a few events that make me smile. As mentioned, we were living in a duplex somehow within the periphery of the oldest, most elegant and statuesque neighborhood in Denver. A typical walk took us past exquisitely designed homes that must have dated back to early 1900's. I have no reference point of eras for great architecture, nor do I make any claims to have extensive knowledge of what constitutes historical design. But. I know that the homes we would walk by were exceptional. I say this to paint a picture of wide neighborhood roads with massive, overhanging mature trees and professionally landscaped gardens. All relatively visible to the passerby.

The homes aligned next to one another. One old mansion sat long on a corner with a huge front yard. The home had a sense of being uncared for, it seemed lonely. Empty. Somehow I must have been privy to a neighborhood tale that there was a young, older man (60's) who lived there alone as his wife had passed and kids were grown. I never saw any 'life' at the home - which was typical because these home owners probably had a dozen homes all over the world.

On a weekend afternoon, within two or three weeks before Keeley's last day, we were on a typical neighborhood stroll. The man stood in the wide, expansive front lawn with a black dog a bit bigger than Keeley. The man looked like his home. Disheveled, but kind. As we walked by, he said hello.

THE END.

The man asked if Keeley would like to say hi. He appeared to be training his dog, as they were on the front lawn with no leash and maybe some sort of a toy to practice fetching. I gave the man my typical response, and assumed he would nod in appreciation of me not setting up his dog for a 'tangle'.

The man said, gently - 'she's fine...she is giving the sign that she wants to play.' I let Keeley off leash, and the two dogs played for maybe 20 minutes. The black dog, I learned, was still a puppy. An Australian Mastiff recently shipped to the states, and then to the new owner. Something about this experience felt so validating. Not validating me, as the owner of Keeley, but validating for Keeley.

There was another neighborhood character that I had befriended. A retired medical doctor that never retired. I wish I could remember the details of his dog story. The man and his Italian greyhound would walk around the neighborhood off leash. We were close to a popular shopping area with a big mall and extended streets that included more shopping, restaurants, coffee shops, etc. Plenty of benches and outdoor patios to sit and people watch. The dog owner had a presence and a certain type of enmeshment with his dog that drew others to them - like street performers. They would sit, and the dog would lay like a scarf around the owner's neck. I would always be awed that this man walked an Italian Greyhound OFF LEASH (the dog looked like it could go from 0 to 60 mph in a SHOT).

Our neighborhood was framed by busy roads. Within the neighborhood, it was quiet and relatively spacious. Still, I was forever scared that Keeley would take off and get hit by a car. Funny how Keeley and I went from this untamed, wild nature to me being a hesitant veer-away-from-all leash walker.

The man and his greyhound walked by my duplex one early evening. My duplex was on the corner of a very busy one way street - 6th avenue. I had a friend from school over, and we were sitting on my front porch. Keeley was inside, and the big front window was open. My friend had a new puppy that was still happy to be on her lap, or under her chair. The man and the off leash Italian-skinny-fast-crazy-disproportionate-long-legs-that-looked-like-it-could-jump-straight-up-20- feet, came onto the porch. He said, 'let her out here' - speaking of Michellie. I'm sure I turned pale. Like, what are you thinking? We are on a corner. He and my relationship was based on me in awe of him walking off leash with his dog, without a care or concern. He had all the confidence in the world that Keeley could manage on the patio. I let her out. She was so happy. No issue.

We drove up to Breckenridge the last weekend she was alive. We had gone for a run before we left, and I forgot to bring water. Keeley was the BEST road trip companion. She had this way of sitting up and looking out the windows at the scenery, as if she was really enjoying herself. She had the slightly open jowl thing going on that looks like a big, happy smile. The traffic sucked, and we ended up backtracking and taking an alternative highway that would take us another three hours. I was going up for a party, and I dropped Keeley off at my friend's house (put out food and water) and then left for the event.

When I got back that evening, I recall letting her out to go to the bathroom and nothing seemed out of the ordinary. The next morning, I got up and drank weekend coffee - I could do this for hours, and it was typical for Keeley to stay sleeping in bed for up to an hour or two after I got out. It had been a long time. I went in to check on her, and she wasn't moving. I picked her up and brought her out to the couch. She was distant, and her gums were white. My best angle was that she was dehydrated. I brought water to her and she did drink.

I managed to get her down the mountain. Once home, I gave her some water with electrolytes. She was laying on my bed. I laid behind her along the length of her. I held her and whispered through the alphabet. Each letter sharing an appreciation of what she meant to me. I distinctly remember the letter 'u'. Us. I love us Keeley. I love what we got to be together.

She actually rebounded and I went to work the next day. When I got home from work, her little heart was still beating too fast, it seemed out of rhythm. I took her to the vet, and the vet said she was good.

The next morning it was back. She moved so slow that I didn't need a leash. I took her out the front to see if she could walk to the corner. She walked to the car and just sat on her hunches by the back passenger side door. I left her to get my keys. She. Unleashed on the corner. I knew I wasn't coming home with her.

It's weird when you think of what this moment would be like. I just knew. Keeley was out. She made the choice. Even when we sat in the garden at the vet. There was no last special moment. She was done. Ready.

After she was dead, the vet said I could stay with her as long as I wanted. It didn't make sense to me. Keeley was part of everything now. I could feel it. She was not in that body.

Somehow I decided that I would just follow the feelings that showed up. I would cry when crying came - wherever and whenever within reason. I made the choice to enjoy the memories, and be happy that I got to have Keeley. It wasn't that I didn't want to feel. Something about the entire experience of Keeley seemed like a gift that was intended to be enjoyed. Always.

Within the next week I moved. I went for a walk.

I met Smoosh.

lesson.

love.

love exists.

Guess who no longer thinks she is a fuck up?

I was just beginning my new journey toward *love* when Keeley died - loving myself enough to recognize that *love* was ever present, an energy. That's not really true. I think we begin the journey back as soon as we come into this physical space.

When I practiced skills, tools, and strategies that aligned with the expansive energy, it felt good. It felt right. I had to care about myself (self-care) enough to be curious. If I could get curious, I could get to the next step. And then the next step. I can assure you that the space grows.

Keeley and I were on Sixth Avenue for two years after the Breckenridge summer. Life events happened that led to a bankruptcy, moving, and Keeley dying all at the same time.

That was over six years ago. I know this because Smoosh turned six earlier this year. Smoosh was just a puppy when I met her the week after I moved to Dakota Ave.

When I walk out my door, the sign across the street reads, 'Unique'. Down from there is a dispensary, 'Livwell'. The corner across from Unique is a sign, 'Goodheart' - a veterinary clinic. Another sign: 'Sally' (beauty supply).

In looking back, it seems a painfully long process to get to my 'shift'. At present, I haven't had an episode in maybe close to three years.

I had the intention of creating online courses the school year AFTER the Breckenridge summer. I quit the full-time job the following school year, and was certain mindfulness was going to be a hit. I was going to create online courses and facilitate workshops.

I got a part-time job at a virtual school which, to me, was all the evidence I needed - 'it' was happening. The virtual school didn't need, nor want, a social-emotional course creator - they wanted a school social worker.

I posted early videos on YouTube of the Check IN that I used at Virtual Academy - my first...technique?

I also created Movement.Breath.Kindness. for elementary classrooms.

My original idea was solid - online course creation and mindfulness as an effective tool to grow social and emotional wellbeing was not lacking in potential. What I didn't realize was that the idea was just that - an idea. A seed. I planted it, and like a nieve gardener, expected results much too soon.

My PhD, or my culminating experience in this particular developmental stage, came in the form of Kung Fu Panda. I was Po. I'll give the five year old (when we met - we hung out for three full years)...I'll give him Master Oogway. Shifu was a beast. We went hip to shoulder for most of his third grade year into half of fourth. A master teacher. The furious five round up all lived on my caseload - each with superhuman powers that transcended common understanding. The setting for the projection of this Kung Fu Panda live action play was Westgate elementary school. It was exactly what I needed to grasp the broad view of not only what it meant to be a school mental health provider, but what it meant to trust *love*.

Po was chosen to be the dragon warrior. The chosen one to bring peace back to the valley. We are all Po. Po was out of tune. Po didn't fit in. Po didn't know his story. Po was clumbsy. Po was 'extra'.

But Po was really good at one thing: being Po.

We are the only one who can bring peace back to our valley.

III

possibility.

She lives in joyful anticipation of the next great thing.

Part three includes a sequence of skills, tools, and strategies that support one's practice of returning to the feeling state of possibility over and over again. The chapters are taken from an online course, self-care, that was created in January 2020. The course was created for school mental health providers to experience the skills in their personal life first; as well as have skills, tools, and strategies to share with their students.

mindfulness.

Grounding feet.

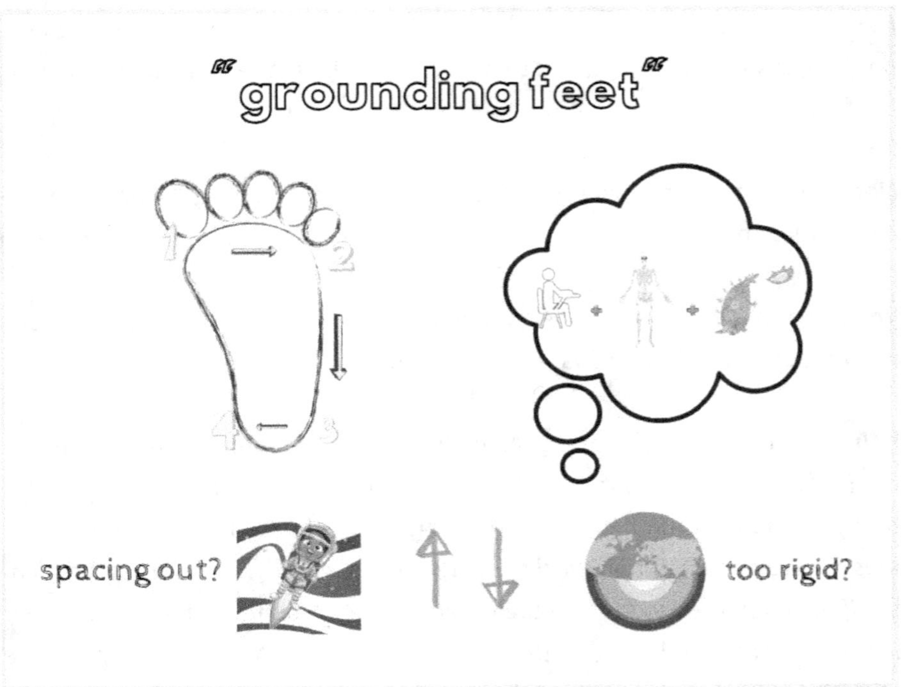

see workbook for more details

Grounding feet is good always. Like everything, it begins with self-awareness (as far as the use of it for self-care). When you care about yourself, you soothe yourself when you notice the feelings of being agitated, or out of sync with the way you like to feel (balanced - not too much, not too little, enough). For those of you familiar with the popular emotional regulation curriculum, Zones of Regulation, this is a great skill when you notice you are in the yellow zone.

This is how I do it and my 'why' - you may have your own interpretation and application.

Bring your awareness to your big toes and push them into the ground (sitting or standing). Notice the sensation (best you can without judgment, comparison, criticism). Then spread your toes out as much as you can and plant your little toe into the ground. In yoga, toe spreading is cued often which is how I learned. Next bring your awareness to the sensation of grounding the back of your heel on the side of the little toe, and then over to the inside back heel, behind your big toe.

Notice the sensation in your feet. Best you can, without judgement, comparison, criticism.

You can end it there. It may be enough to bring you back to present moment awareness and feeling in charge of your focus.

***In the slide I have a thought bubble. When I prepare a class or small group for a mindfulness practice, I tell them to notice where they are in space and time. I also add, 'notice what it's like to be exactly who you are...now.' I desire to get kids curious about their physical body sitting in a balanced way by having them see if they can be curious about their skeleton - their bones. Is the left and right side of their body in balance if they could see their skeleton in an xray? Is there space between the bones? In the slide, the dragon icon represents breath. <u>Notice where you are in space and time. Are you sitting in a way that feels balanced: not too much, not too little, enough. Breathe. Notice breath in your body.</u>*

Here is a little more understanding for your own application, or to facilitate for others:

Consider left brain and right brain. Left brain being in charge of right side of body, and right brain being in charge of left side of the body. When we feel out of sync with balance it is because we ARE out of balance. You may have a concrete understanding of balance as it relates to motor skills and vestibular sensation in reference to students, or your self (ie. vertigo). Take a second to just wonder about your emotional balance on the inside – not too much, not too little, enough. What does enough feel like? You have a way of being exactly who you are. You have a guidance mechanism inside of you, your intuition. It doesn't go anywhere. We just disconnect ourselves from it. It will lead you if you allow it to. If you aren't familiar with it, the more you are curious and the more you practice awareness of your inside world, you naturally resonate with what you call intuition, your knowing. It's your thing. Between you and you.

When we get out of sync with balance, we tend to do one of two things (generally speaking). We get super rigid or super spacey. Our awareness and the skill of notice.name. (check IN) can help us recognize where we may be stuck. We can use our breath, and our imagination, to bring us back to a more integrated, balanced, experience of present moment.

Feeling spacey? Ground yourself into the physical space by imagining yourself breathing in all that spacey from above (non physical space, not something you can interpret through your 5 physical senses), breathe it in through the crown of your head, through your body, down through your feet into the ground. Ground the spacey energy as you breathe out. Notice the experience. Name the sensation of the experience – best you can. Allow the experience by observing rather than judging, comparing, critiquing. By noticing, naming, and allowing, the energy that isn't helpful can move through and release. Your cells want to be balanced, they know how to get there. Give them space to do their thing.

Feeling rigid? Breathe in the physical ground energy (use your imagination to draw it up from inside the earth) and send it to the space above as you breathe out, and then breathe in the space above and send it to the earth as you breathe out.

If you are ambidextrous enough to imagine the left side and the right side - go for it and breathe in space down through the left side of your brain into the right side of your body, into the earth. Then breathe up the ground energy up through the left side of the body, up through the right side of your brain and into space above. I attend yoga nidra, I have never studied it. I think nidra supports this concept - integrating energy in one's body through breath.

Practice on your own self. Care about yourself to be curious how to soothe your nervous system and responses (impulses/urges). Once you understand how it works and experience the soothing sensation in your own body, it is easy to share with others. And actually, when you do share with others, your own understanding and practice grows even more. Funny how that works.

*** At the time this was written, I had a real time experience of a student in 4th grade who lived in his right brain, spacey, most of the time at school (he was also quite overwhelmed at school so there was the element of escape). Every time I met with him we practiced grounding feet. It wasn't pretty. He was highly distracted. He got better each time, and I learned a lot about what and why I was facilitating the skill for him. I was not attached to a specific outcome, I chose to stay curious. Sometimes I felt like an idiot, but I figured I would know when it was time to move on. As soon as you think you are off track is when the student, parent, or teacher makes some comment about the student using the skill effectively. It hadn't happened yet in this scenario. I personally used the skill on an airplane that was delayed - once boarded - for 2 hours. It worked perfectly and got me into focus to work on this project.*

5 senses.

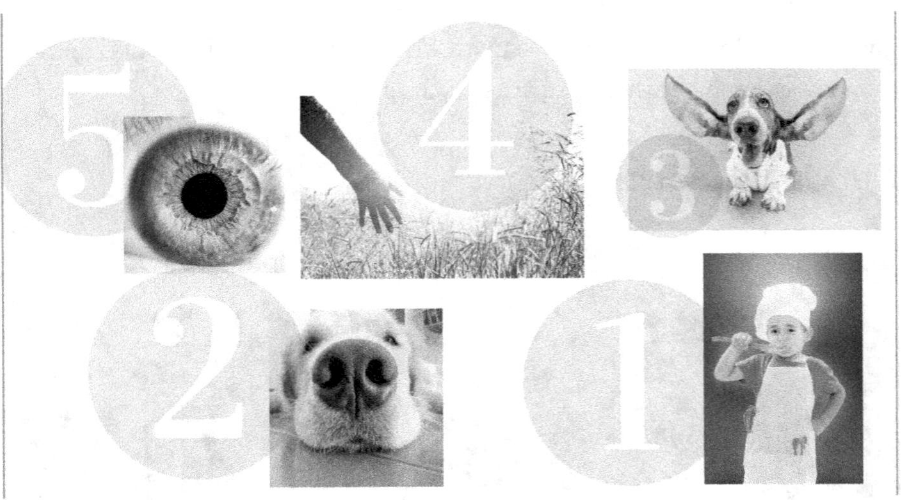

5 senses is a standard mindfulness practice - I think it is a skillset that is part of Jon Kabat Zinn's popular and research based, Mindfulness Based Stress Reduction (MBSR). Most mindfulness practices that were used 8 years ago when I first got interested in teaching it to others were MBSR techniques.

Notice and name. 5 senses. Begin by noticing and naming 5 things that you see. Best you can without judgement, comparison, or criticism. I say to the student to be a curious observer of their experience as if they are a scientist. Notice and name 4 felt sensations in physical space and time (clothing, ground, chair, etc). 3 sounds. 2 smells. 1 taste. Invite in your own calming experience of the senses if it makes more 'sense' (ha). The object is to ground your energy into present time and space by bringing awareness to physical senses, soothing the nervous system to have choice around focus.

Self-awareness is the gateway to this skill being integrated throughout your day. Someone asked me what I do for self-care, and I thought to myself – 'what don't I do?' . Once you notice you are out of alignment, out of sync – implement a strategy and anticipate the outcome of balance and a return to you being in charge of focus. The more you practice, it becomes a habit and you continually practice – constantly returning to balance and present moment awareness where you are in charge of focus.

Noticing sensations.

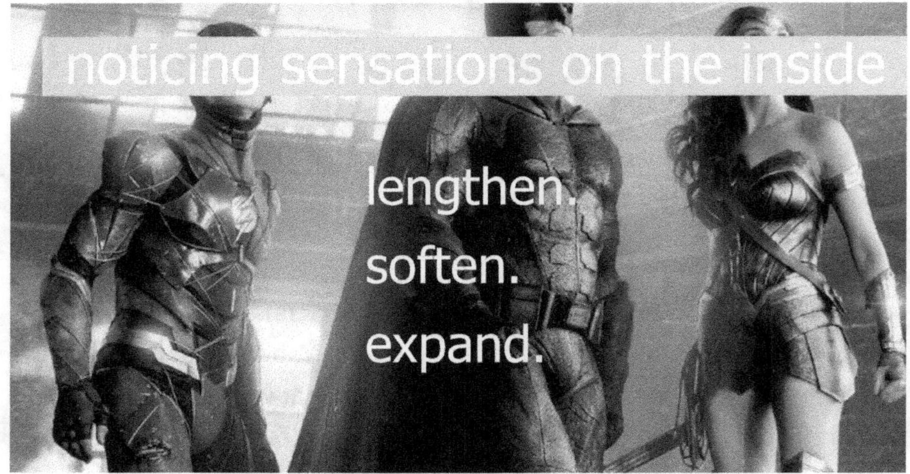

Sensations were really tricky for me when I first began practicing and facilitating mindfulness. It took me a long time to get mindful because I was so easily distracted and I wanted knowledge. My morning mindfulness practice began with coffee and reading. And then I found things to listen to online. I had a lot of momentum in thinking and gaining knowledge, and considering how I was going to teach what I was learning to others....rather than having the experience, and being a curious observer of experience, without the attachment to particular outcomes. I also did not like it when an author, or person I was being influenced by, told me some version of 'it's not easy', 'it takes work', 'you have to do the work'. I think there is a balance in that overall. I did do a HELL of a lot of personal work. I also feel that my most desired outcome was to understand the skills so that I could facilitate it to others in a simple way. I think it took me a long time because of the level of understanding and experience I wanted to have as a facilitator. I don't think results need to take that long – and that we 'earn' outcomes, and it should be hard to be worthwhile. I think life is meant to be enjoyed – now.

Sensations. Lengthen something. Notice the sensation of lengthening. Can you be curious about the sensation? Soften something. Notice the sensation of softening. Can you be curious about the sensation? Comfortable or uncomfortable? Too much or not enough? Expand. Expand something. Notice the sensation of expansion. Can you be curious about the sensation?

Easy application: sitting or standing – lengthen spine, soften shoulders, expand chest (heart space). Do this throughout the day. Notice the reset. It becomes a habit.

Amy Cuddy's popular TED talk can be great here – as this slide tees up the superhero pose. Amy also has an awesome book, *Presence,* that I couldn't stop listening to on my Audible app.

tips.

A few years ago, I was asked to facilitate a 20-minute presentation on *How to Motivate and Inspire Students* for staff professional development. Honestly, if I could master this topic to a group of overburdened and underappreciated elementary school teachers in 20 minutes then I am an educational prophet.

I created at least a 60-minute presentation that I attempted to fit into 20 minutes.

I titled my presentation *Inspired to Inspire*, and shared relevant tools and strategies that supported awareness and growth of what I consider to be the top three skills to grow wellbeing: self-awareness, sensory processing/integration, and emotional regulation.

moving forward, let's define wellbeing as a general state of balance (a sense of equilibrium - not too much, not too little, enough)

How does one inspire anyone else if one is not inspired? One cannot access an inspired state if one is not regulated.

As I spent a ridiculous amount of time preparing for the presentation, I narrowed down three practice tips (skills) that help when presenting personal material to a general audience who may or may not want to be receiving what you are sharing.

This hard-to-read slide (that I happen to have become quite fond of) includes a more recent interpretation of the three practice tips that support audience engagement.

three helpful practice tips

RECOGNIZE RESISTANCE	ON BOARD THINKING	CHOOSE CURIOUS
notice how you respond to a new idea.	what CAN you get 'on board' with...	choosing an attitude or state of curiosity allows access to problem solving (executive functions/higher order thinking skills)
open sensation - not threatened	"I may not agree with ________, but I can be open to__________."	
closed sensation - potential threat		"I wonder why____"
recognizing your state allows you to choose.		"Why am I______"
		"What if _____"

How are these tools relevant as you practice self-care?

1. <u>Recognizing Resistance.</u> If you only learned how to use the skill of self-awareness* to become aware of resistance, you have placed yourself in the driver's seat for positive change as it relates to day-to-day satisfaction of your ordinary experience. Resistance is what keeps us from moving toward discomfort. Resistance can feel like a tight tummy, an urge to argue, a repeated monologue, a headache, quitting, etc.

Resistance is a wall that separates you from possibility. In a simple way, resistance is the stress response. The stress response (fight, flight, freeze, faint) is a highly intelligent system of protection. When the stress response is triggered we can consider ourselves to be in a closed state because we become rote. We survive. Our brain stem and limbic system are on auto pilot and the ability to thoughtfully choose to move toward a potential danger, threat, or challenge (perception of the problem) and be a problem solver is shut down. In school language, we cut ourselves off from our executive skills. We can learn all we want about executive skills – but they can't be accessed if we are not regulated (in a balanced state).

2. <u>On Board Thinking</u>. I love that I came up with this term. Actually, I don't know if I originated it or not - probably not and it really doesn't matter. It is such a great term for those of us who visualize. It is also a fabulous 'piggy-back' to Recognizing Resistance. When you catch resistance, the resistance can be slowed by validating your response (okay I am not on board with ___________) and ask yourself, 'what CAN I get on-board with?' If I'm at yoga practice and the instructor says something that I don't agree with - do I get up and leave or have a miserable yoga practice - NO. I catch the resistance and tell my own story that soothes my nervous system and supports my alignment with possibility.

3. <u>Choose Curious</u>. These three shared skills, or 'tips', are meant to be very accessible and practical. Each of these skills can include so much more depth for understanding. To keep this simple, when I Choose Curious I am asking questions in a thoughtful way. If I am asking a question, I have set myself up to receive an answer. As we develop skills, we can learn to allow. Curiosity is the gateway to accessing higher order thinking - the open state where a broader view lives (*executive skills* in school speak).

*I use the terms mindfulness and self-awareness interchangeably.

brainstorm.

Post-Dated Journal Entry

The Post-Dated Journal Entry is not an original concept. It is exactly what it sounds like it is: choose a segment of time, and post date a journal entry that you would write as if everything is happening exactly how you wish - on that future date.

I mentioned the summer that I went to Breckenridge for June and July. I post-dated a journal entry for August 1 that I created on June 1. I read the journal entry every morning, and created the 'state' of what it would be like to really be living the manifested reality. Totally worked. However, it did not sustain itself because I had not developed the skillsets, or understanding, of what I was actually doing. I had lost 20 pounds in two months, and had great energy. I found a fun place to live that I moved into on Labor Day. Keeley (my dog) who had broken her paw a day before we left for the mountains, had no sign of breakage on the xray at her next vet visit and was able to hike and play outside within a week or two after it happened. I fit into everything I ever bought (I had a habit of buying clothes that I was GOING to fit into). I even became great friends with a woman who owned her own coffeeshop and baked all her own pastries (we are still friends to this day...that was not necessarily on my Post-Dated Journal Entry, but I was always daydreaming of working at a coffeeshop).

Eight years ago, the manifested desires were all external things that I thought would make me happy once I attained them. I now realize that you make yourself happy by regulating your energy, noticing your thinking patterns, and telling your own story - living in an intentional state of positive expectation. The external desires show up because they align with the state you create by caring about how you feel moment to moment. As these ideas develop, the concepts will make more sense. Stick with it. There is a reason you are engaging in this book.

Get a notebook. Open a document on your computer. And get.after.it. As you practice, you may start to create in small segments. For example, on a Sunday night you may consider the following Sunday night. What makes a great Sunday night? Beginning with the end in mind. (BTW...I love Leader in Me which is a school social-emotional curriculum based on Stephen Covey's 7 habits of highly effective people. All wellbeing skills, tools, and strategies can be channeled through the program. I worked at several Leader in Me schools and gradually integrated all my ideas into Covey's framework. Genius).

post-dated journal entry

Choose a segment of time and post date a journal entry that you would write as if everything is happening exactly how you wish - on that date.
'I am so happy now that...'

Creative Visualization

As mentioned, I met a new friend in Breckenridge during 'the summer of change' who was transitioning from being a full-time mental health therapist, to being the owner of a coffeeshop. On a side note, it may be of interest to mention that working in a coffeeshop was my fantasy when things got overwhelming (which was often). Anyway, she had boxes of books stored in her garage. I think that was where I found a copy of Shatki Gawain's *Creative Visualization.*

I used Shatki's chapter on Setting Goals as a strategy to *create* a desire for more. The reason I italicized the word *create* is because that is the skill being developed when we brainstorm new ideas and possibilities.

When I first got into this content area of self-development and personal growth, I thought I was on board with visualization. The concept of visualizing made sense to me. If you have ever been an athlete or interested in sports or performance in general, it is commonly understood that elite athletes and/or performers use visualization as a tool for top performance. Visualize the outcome you desire. Take in the sensory experience of the desired outcome – the feel of your body, the roar of the crowd, etc. This made and makes sense to me.

When I intentionally began to use this skill, I found that it was not as easy as I assumed. When you *create*, by using your imagination, new outcomes and the sensory experience and details of those new outcomes, you are creating new neural pathways. By virtue of this being a new or underdeveloped pathway, you are designing it as if it doesn't exist or at least the familiarity of the pathway is not available. As easy as it seems to *create* desired outcomes, it does take some focus to get started on new 'visions'. It also can be difficult in the early stages as those around you may not be on board with your new desires. Depending on the novelty of your idea (think Steve Jobs) you are creating new pathways that are not familiar to those who spend the most time with you, which can make relationships a bit uncomfortable. People have familiar pathways of relating to you and others in general (as humans we don't always do well with unexpected behavior – especially with people we have known for a long time). Let's not get too into the 'others' yet. Self-care is caring about yourself. The use and development of skills, tools, and strategies that grow your wellbeing is between you and you.

Shatki's brainstorming activity can support the experience of creating. Get on board by considering the development of the skill: to *create*. Notice discomfort, and see if you can intentionally move toward the discomfort with a desire to shift into a fun, playful (creative) state by using the skill of creating that lives in the prefrontal cortex where fun and playfulness can be accessed. Notice the self-talk. A popular resource that I often came across in my own process was called 'the Artist's Way' by Julia Cameron. I never completed the course, but I did begin it and recall Julia's discussion about 'the blurt'. She talked about listening for the blurt and *flipping the blurt*, or being curious about the blurt. The blurt is the inner voice that can sound like self-doubt. For example, when you brainstorm your desires, you may limit your capacity to *create* by listening to the blurt that suggests that your desire is immoral, unconventional, impractical, etc. Self-awareness helps you notice the blurt and *flip the blurt*: : 'what if I can________', 'what if it was true', etc.

When we get stuck, or find ourselves spinning, in life results that never seem quite satisfying, we are most likely operating from the well worn neural pathways of familiarity. Whether or not these pathways are helpful or hurtful is not necessarily something we tend to consider. Outcomes are familiar (we have seen, smelled, tasted, touched this before) and the patterns continue to stay deeply embedded, until we become aware of the patterns that limit us and intentionally disrupt them.

To become aware of the patterns is the only place to begin. But then what? Here is where our capacity, and innate skill, to *create* new outcomes becomes quite relevant. Once you recognize the thinking pattern (belief, mindset, paradigm) that is limiting you, you want to disrupt the pattern by telling a new story. We are living in the age of disruption (politics, retail, transportation, media, entertainment, etc). It is cool to disrupt.

Practicing tools that support creating new ideas helps us to grow new neural pathways, and get out of the familiar well worn pathways that limit us.

I am <u>not one</u> to set goals as much as I <u>am one</u> to set goals. I tend to set themes and reasonable expectations for segments of time. I also like to *create* or write stories about my life unfolding in fun and fabulous ways. What the stories are creating is a state of positive expectation, which allows me to enjoy the journey and the moment rather than be attached to, and obsessed with, a particular outcome. I return to this reminder often as I *create* this sequence of skills. Obviously there is an outcome to publish. The joy (to enjoy) is now. The process. The journey.

This brainstorm activity may just be that – a brainstorm activity that supports your ability to *create* new ideas and outcomes. Creating is a skill, an ability. Everyone has it. Below are slides from a recent lesson to middle school students where I facilitated my own version Shatki's activity. I also used the activity straight from the book in the original course I taught to high school students.

CREATIVE VISUALIZATION

Keeping in mind your present life situation, write down under each of the following categories some things that you would like to have, to change, or to improve upon in the NEAR future. Don't think about it too hard; simply write down any ideas that come to your mind as good possibilities.

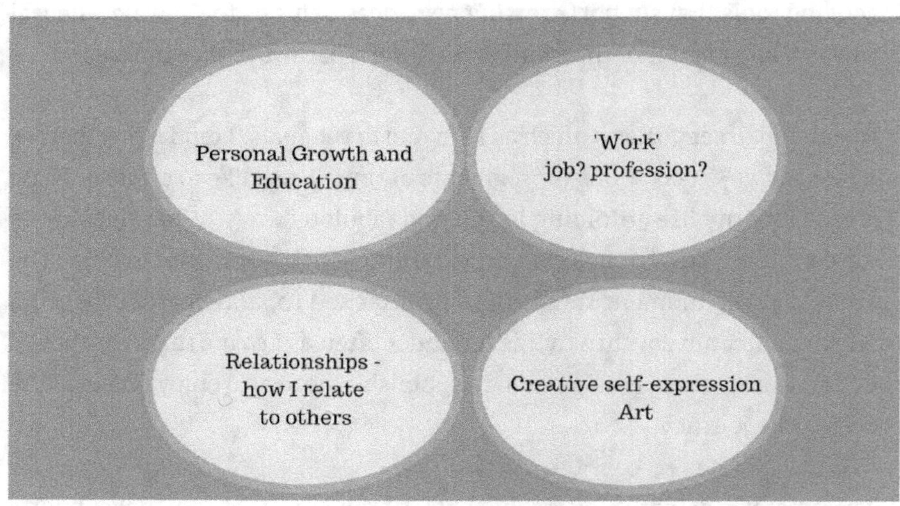

Personal Growth and Education
'Work' job? profession?
Relationships - how I relate to others
Creative self-expression Art

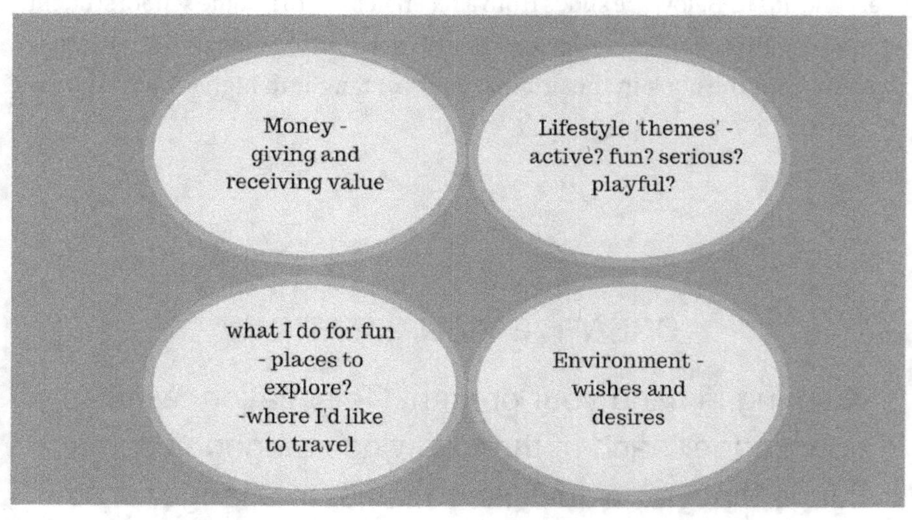

Money - giving and receiving value
Lifestyle 'themes' - active? fun? serious? playful?
what I do for fun - places to explore? -where I'd like to travel
Environment - wishes and desires

CREATIVE VISUALIZATION - PART TWO

Now...for fun and practice using your creativity and imagination...brainstorm ENDLESS possibilities...if ANYTHING were possible...what would you desire to be, do, or have in ANY category.

Writing Prompt

The outcome of this activity is to have the experience of using your innate skill to *create*, and to enjoy the fun and playful 'state' that creating preferred outcomes brings. Notice the 'blurt' and *flip the blurt* (this is a great skill to acquire). *What if I can?*

This writing prompt I return to over and over again. I may do it in my mind while I'm on a walk ,or driving. I love to write. I have multiple notebooks. I write present thoughts that are either curious, positive, fun, validating, or generally uplifting. I write stories that are either funny, or about life as I dream it up and want it to be. Knowing that I am growing the state of possibility, as opposed to being absolutely attached to a specific outcome.

As I reflect, I think my current writing comes from me already being in a state of possibility, or in alignment, with my most balanced, natural state. This means that I do not use my journal writing, or love of writing, to get to the balanced state. I use other skills, tools, and strategies that support the state of possibility, and allow me to get clear (I think it's called meditation - wink wink). I write from that state. This may or may not be true for you.

My current journal writing is the opposite of how it was when I first began in my teen years. I used to be quite proud of the pages I could fill up in a notebook during one sitting. I collected those notebooks, and my collection had grown to quite a number.

When I began graduate school, my 'depression' really showed up full force. I have an experience that is relevant to journaling, and may be relevant to you. Christian Molidor. Christian was the dean of the Graduate School of Social Work when I began the program. I didn't have him as a professor, and I'm not sure how we began our interactions. I think his office was near one of my classes, and I would say hi to him and stop to talk.

In one discussion, I must have mentioned the depression. Christian was an LCSW, and you know how those 'therapist-types' are...it gets real - fast. I think he inquired about the depression, and asked if I journaled. I felt as if a spotlight came on, I had this opportunity to really shine in front of this human I wanted to impress (by virtue of his status in the program). What a perfect question setting me up to look good.

Of course I told him all the amazing journaling I had done, and all the notebooks that I had kept and just happened to have all in one box, as I had just moved to Denver. He said, 'why don't you bring in a few notebooks and maybe I can understand your thinking a bit and we can work on this 'depression.' Something like that - it was fall of 2005, my memory isn't all that great for detail.

I felt special that the dean of the GSSW was open to spending time with me. In preparation for our meeting, I thought I should look at my journals to have a peek at what he may be seeing. When I 'peeked' I was astounded at the negativity, and the momentum of the same story over and over. The theme would be hate. I hated myself.

This was the very beginning of graduate school in a clinical field. I was by no means any sort of expert in understanding human behavior (I thought I was - that's another story). I picked up on the pattern fast and could not be free of those notebooks any faster. It was as if they literally caught on fire. I hurled them out away from me as quickly as I could. Ew. No more.

I stopped journaling.

As I write this and am reflecting, I think I began journaling again to kick off the Breckenridge summer. I have no recollection of notebooks prior to that time.

I can think back to things I said, did, or wondered about long before I began getting curious about enlightenment or self-care, personal growth, etc. We are constantly connecting to our highest self long before we have labeled or categorized our thinking, giving it a hashtag, and making meaning of it. I was ignorant, and out of sync, with so much that I understand now; but I knew enough to stop the harmful pattern I had created.

Without a coach or a therapist, I had a very clear introspection that writing in detail about how much I hated myself was not the answer. It was actually the opposite. Hating myself was the antithesis to what I desired.

The writing prompt that I currently use is simple. Once again, it is definitely not my original concept as you may already be familiar with it.

You choose:: 'If' or 'Since' I can be, do, or have ANYTHING without money, time, or other resources being of concern or limitation, what do I desire?

Practice tips to consider:
- remember a curiosity about 'the blurt' - skill: flip the blurt
- self-care (caring about yourself) mindset or attitude: it's between you and you.

Remember, the end game (that never ends) is to *create*. To be curious. To wonder. To expand. These are all skillsets and states that align with the field of possibility. You may notice that the skills, tools, and strategies I am sharing are all resources to align you with the most natural and balanced version of you. That's it. What you do and where you go from there? You *create* your content. You tell your story.

mission.

This is a fun activity that I did recently with middle school students. I can't remember where I got this original idea. I do remember when I did the activity for the first time, and LOVING the idea behind it (I don't want to give it away). It was a fun surprise that you only get the first time you do it. Make sure you set up the activity with enough time if you facilitate to students. Otherwise, they miss the fun of discovery.

Here are images of the 'Now Introducing' slides with examples. If you are doing this just for self-care, use a notebook. I continue to use this practice when I feel the need to reflect and get centered. I like the discovery of what character attributes I am attracting, or curious about.

this activity is created to reflect and respond to the uplifting, life-giving, and positive influences that are relevant in your life as you are experiencing it in the now...not influences that are triggering or upsetting.

1. List 5 influential people, ideas, or things relevant to your life right now.

2. Now write at least one quality for each choice that really stands out.

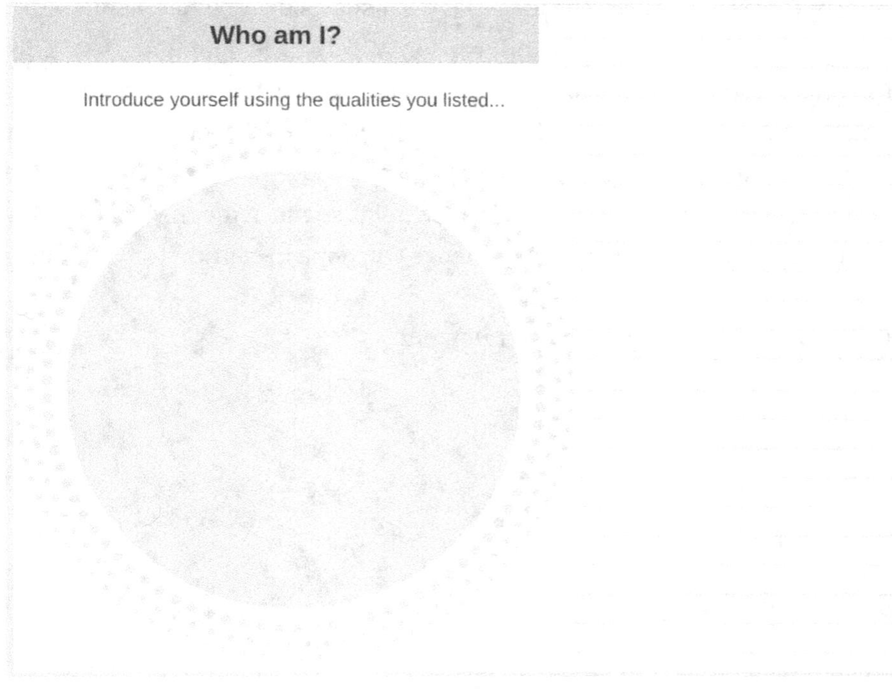

see example in appendix

When I presented this activity to middle schoolers, I referred to it as a 'self-branding' exercise and connected it to social media. I challenged them to consider their values and what is meaningful to them as they get curious about 'who am I' and 'how do I desire to show up and express myself'.

I use this activity often for reflection. You may use it to discover what you value. It's interesting what you find of value in others is what you hold true to yourself, or what you desire more of for yourself. When I first began doing this, 'confidence' always came up. I recognized that I value, or am attracted to, confidence in others, yet it was something I was lacking. The activity helped me recognize that confidence was something to focus on growing. Introducing yourself as if you already hold all the attributes, allows you to create the story of you as if it is already happening.

Stephen Covey introduced the idea that what shows up, or what manifests in physical form, is always the second creation. We create in our minds first. This really makes sense when you get curious about it. You don't just act and then something randomly appears..if you think about building a house or growing a garden (easy to see twice creation in these examples). The character attributes also capture the sensory experience which holds so much more when it comes to visualizing, and sensing the experience you hope to capture for yourself.

Here is the second part: mission statement.

Ask yourself...

What breaks my heart?

What makes me feel most alive?

How do I desire to show up and express myself?

Create a mission statement by declaring a statement that combines your greatest heartbreak and your greatest joy.

see example in appendix

This activity supported my mission statement that I have used for at least the last three years. With students, you may just use the activity as a brainstorm, and tease out a mission statement. One student raised his hand and asked me for help. He had written, 'my parents getting a divorce' for 'what breaks my heart'. We considered the theme beneath parents splitting up, and came up with what breaks his heart is change, or when things change. What he loved was video games - play, a challenge. We didn't come up with a mission statement as we ran out of time, but maybe it could have been something like: 'James' sees change as a challenge and uses his love of play to move toward it.' Obviously, the statement needs to resonate with the human creating it - that's the ultimate goal, to create a feeling statement - a statement that empowers.

roles.

I named this next practice 'Broad View' as a title to publish. I think I had been referring to it as '6 roles'.

This 'Broad View' strategy is something that I began doing on my own as a way to create inner space, or to gain perspective when I recognized that I was obsessed with one thing - and, in my case, that one thing was my job. To be obsessed with something you are enjoying is one thing. To be obsessed with something that isn't bringing you joy, is a whole other thing.

How this strategy looked in the day-to-day: when I recognized I was overwhelmed (skill: self-awareness) I would take out my journal, or anything to write on, including a napkin at a coffee shop or the corner of any piece of paper I had access to (at home, I always have 2-3 notebooks going at a time). I would scratch out a horizon line with six sections. Over time, I added the 'now this is me' (mind space, heart space, belly space) picture in the center, which gave the illusion of me looking out into the broad, infinite space of a horizon.

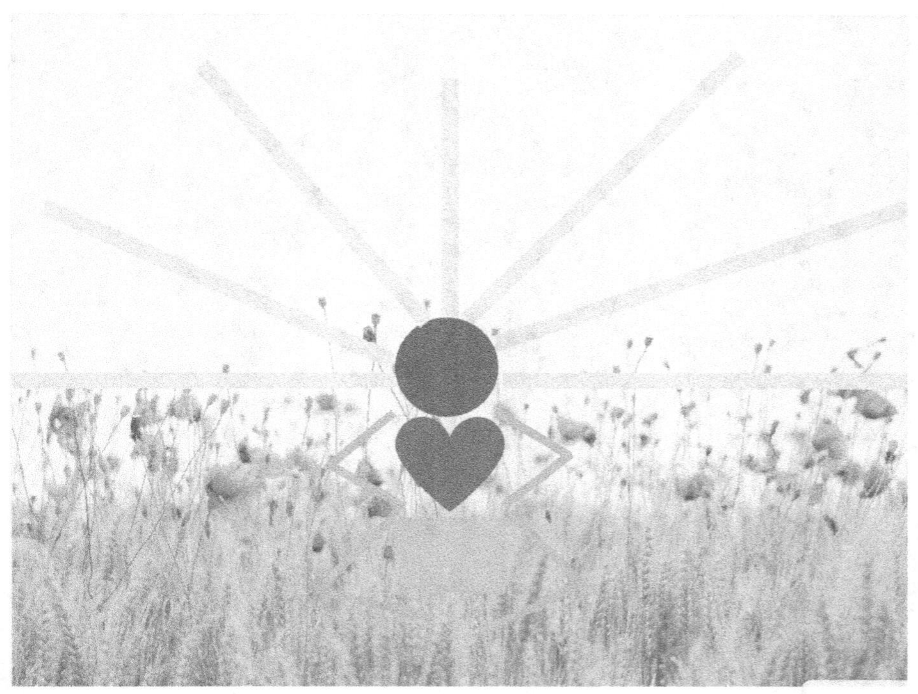

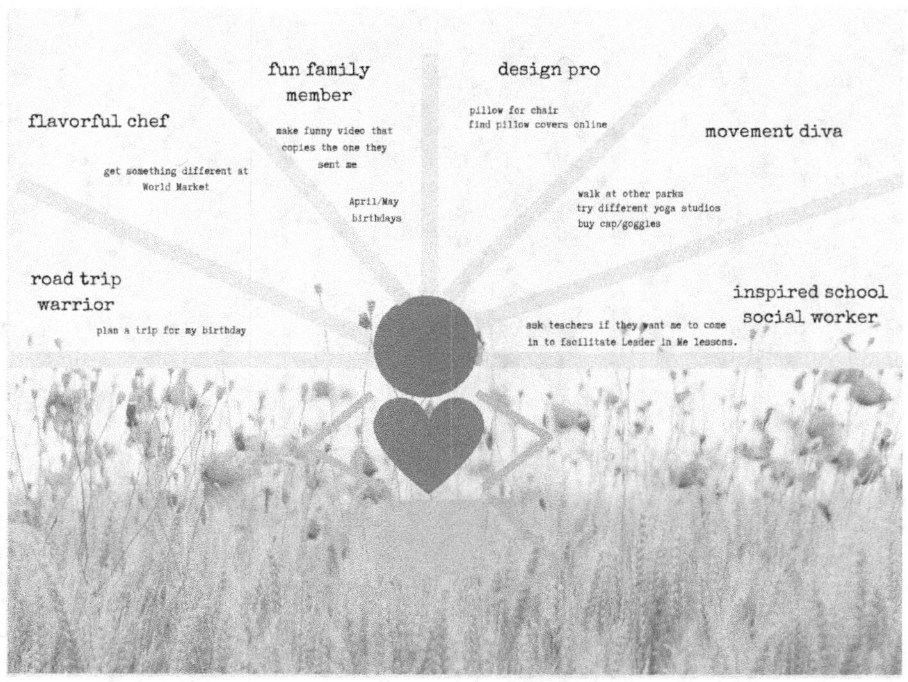

I give each of the six spaces a 'role.'

**I had taken the time to consider my roles when I created a Best Year Yet plan years back, using the strategy Jinny Ditzler created in the 90's. It is a great activity if you are really into self-reflection. The Best Year Yet plan suggests eight roles, and uses that number based on some sort of algorithm-ish of business executives who manage teams. When I took the time to consider my roles, I came up with ways to describe the roles that added some expression, some texture, some visceral interpretation of the roles (think 'radiant goddess' - yep...or something like that).

It seems, like with all things, that you can consider your roles at length, with a lot of reflection, as easily as you can write down the first six that come to you. And, obviously, you can always return to the thought, 'hm. what are six roles that I desire to play out?' – life is fluid as are the roles you choose to focus on. My roles are different today as I write this.

When you name the roles, and create the horizon, randomly fill in what you want more of in each section. In practice, I place the role I am obsessed with on the bottom, and I really don't give it much attention. When I bring focus to the roles I am not actively engaging with, that's when this strategy begins to support expansion, and a more balanced perspective.

*This works as a doodle in long meetings or workshops that can begin to feel overwhelming...as do the other skills like Recognizing Resistance, On-Board Thinking, and Choose Curious.

frame.

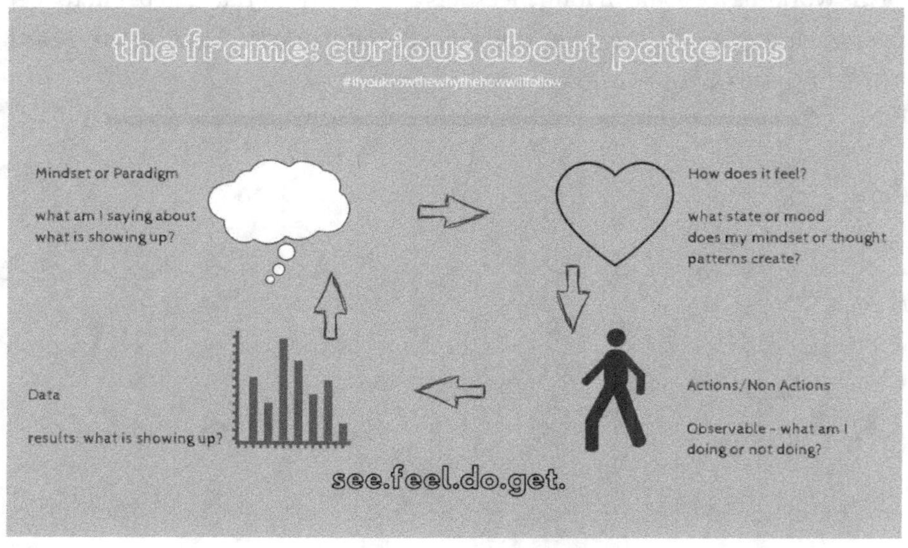

I learned *the frame* during my first year as a school social worker. I attended a two-day training for the social-emotional curriculum, Top Twenty Teens.

I recall being at the training, and feeling like I was exactly where I was supposed to be. I loved it. The training was somehow very personal, and aligned with self-improvement, as much as it was an opportunity to experience and learn skills, tools, and strategies that could be transferred to the students I was working with.

It was the 2007-08 school year when I attended the training. I am fairly certain that I was not thinking growth outcomes, or transferable skills. I did want to teach the kids skills. Obviously, it's easiest to teach the skills that resonate. *The frame* resonated…it made sense. But this was several years before the big epiphany I mentioned in the introduction and the 'why?'.

I have an entirely different approach to *the frame* now. I find *the frame* useful to disrupt limiting thought patterns or beliefs.

The following is taken from a blog post that captured *the frame* @ sallyseifferco.blog:

We can tie together a few of our practices as we examine the usefulness of *the frame* in our ordinary, day-to-day experience.

Start here.

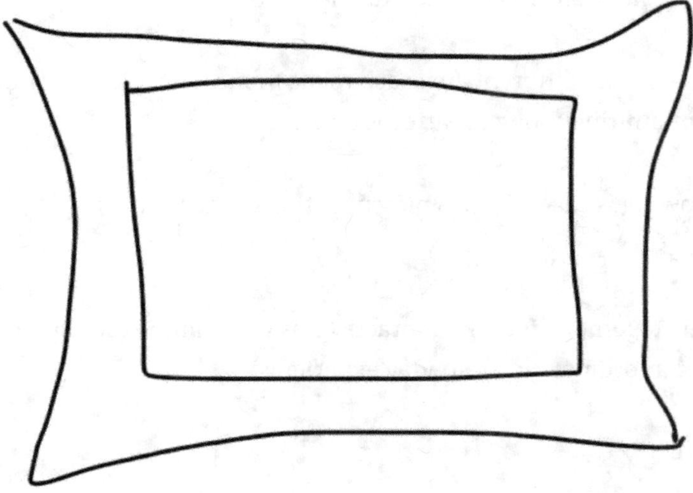

the frame.

Considering the 'picture' you choose…what do you say about the picture? What is your mindset, paradigm, belief (the story you tell) about the circumstance, situation, or event?

When we are practicing self-care, or caring for ourself, it's best to practice new skills, tools, and strategies with general intentions. The goal may be to understand how the new skill, tool, or strategy works. What this means, is that it may not be useful to apply new learning, or ideas, to your most difficult life event, situation, or circumstance.

To practice using *the frame*, choose one of your roles from the '6 roles' or 'Broad View' practice. Choose a role that you have the least resistance to.

What does this role look, feel, sound like - capture the essence of this role as you imagine it inside your frame. We are going to integrate the picture in the frame with 'get'. What results, or data, is showing up in this area of your life? What are you GETting?

75

How do you 'see' the situation, circumstance, event? Hint: the 'story you tell' has a theme.

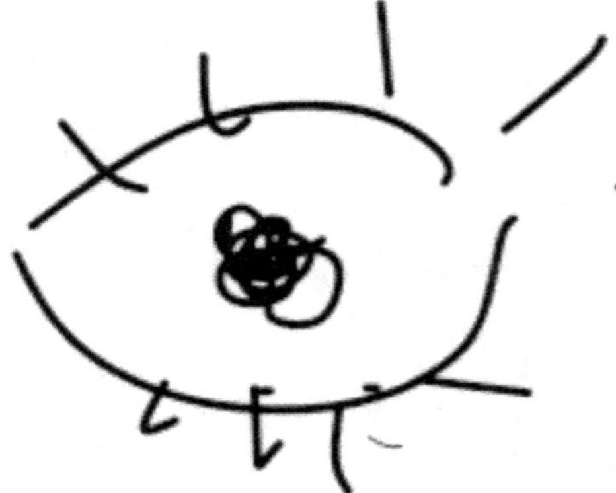

see.

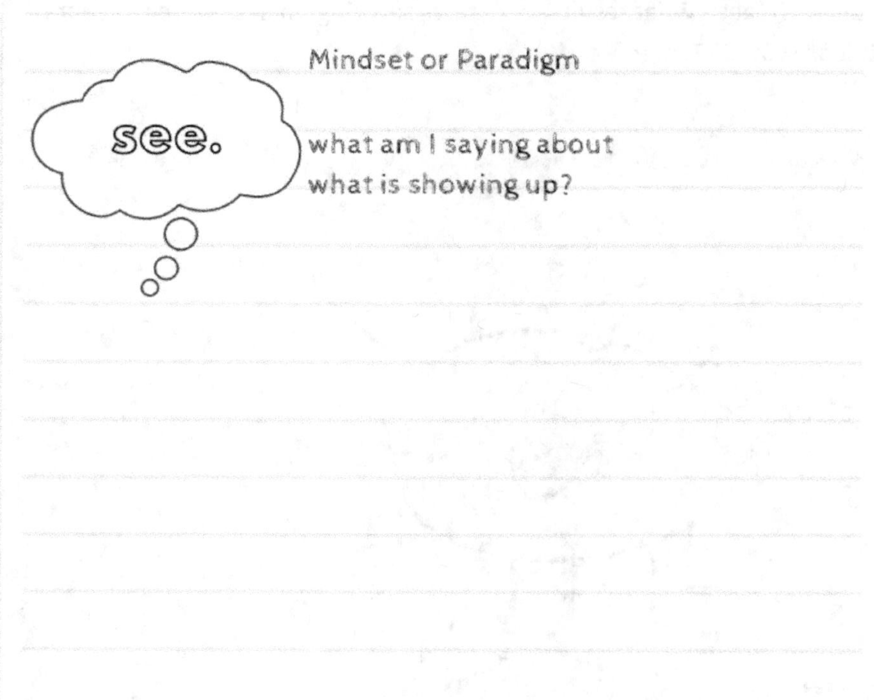

If I were to see a picture of a road trip in my current life experience, it would be non existent. I would see a picture of my metallic grey subaru outback, and I would see the Apple CarPlay with the Audible app and maybe my variety of music apps. I would actually get excited. I love road trips. However, the results – my data (my 'get') is that I haven't been on one in several years. What am I saying about road trips? "I love road trips." The energy is a bit elusive. The road trip is something that is out in front of me, it is *going to* happen some day. I suppose if my mindset is that it's *going to* happen...then it's always kind of hanging out there...I'm *going to* do it at some point. As I examine my 'see' a bit more, I learn that I may see the 'road trip' as 'fluff'. The road trip is not as important as staying in Denver, and working on this project. When this project is complete, THEN I can go on a road trip. If I go on a road trip, I won't have time to work on this project.

I tend to get a bit consumed with things. For me, the reason I created the 6 roles/Broad View is exactly for this reason. If my desire is to enjoy myself now, not in this elusive future state once I get the really important stuff done, then I need to be curious about these different areas of my life and the roles I desire to play.

My 'see' needs to change to 'I can plan a road trip.' Or some version of 'it's happening now' v. it will happen when other more important things get done.

The theme, the 'story you tell', is connected to a 'state' – a mood or a feeling.

feel.

How does it feel?

what state or mood does my mindset or
thought patterns create?

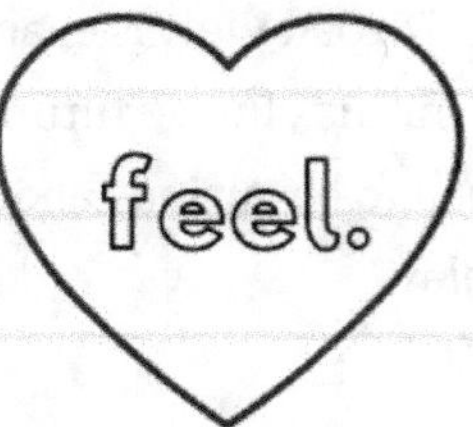

I like considering road trips. When I have felt overwhelmed and practiced 6 roles, considering road trips created a sense of fun, and I suppose a bit of escape. A road trip is an adventure. A road trip is something to look forward to. Positive expectation. The anticipation of something fun happening.

Your 'state' (mood, energy in motion – emotion, feeling...drives behavior – action). The behavior, what you choose to do or not do, is observable. This is where it gets confusing in 'real' life. When we don't take time to slow down, we just observe behavior and react to it. It creates a sense of 'others in charge' and that power is external rather than an internal state (the feeling of empowerment).

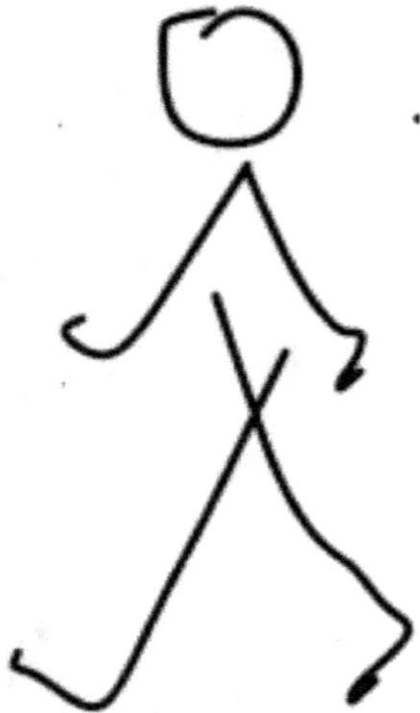

do. (or don't do)

<u>Actions/Non Actions</u>

Observable – what am I
doing or not doing?

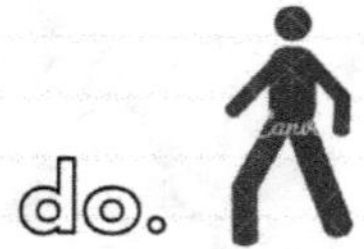

The action here would be to plan. This is where focus comes in handy. When I create a time to focus on planning a road trip, all of a sudden the road trip becomes a reality. I am currently only considering road trips when I practice 6 roles. I have been consumed with this project, so I haven't really considered the reality of a road trip. My action is to create time to plan a road trip. In my journaling, a story I would write begins: She loves to plan road trips. (and yes, the word 'plan' can be elusive...let's not overthink this...because really, the feeling of positive expectancy is enough).

<u>Data</u>

results: what is showing up?

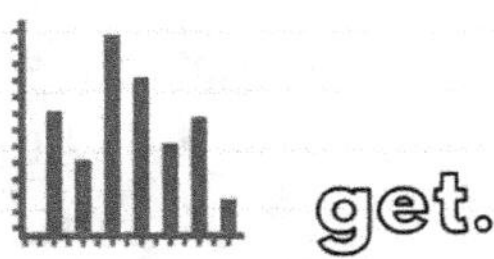

Our action or non action drives our own data — the results that show up in our lives. What we 'get'.

The observable results, the 'get' reinforces the story we tell ("See! I told you!!").

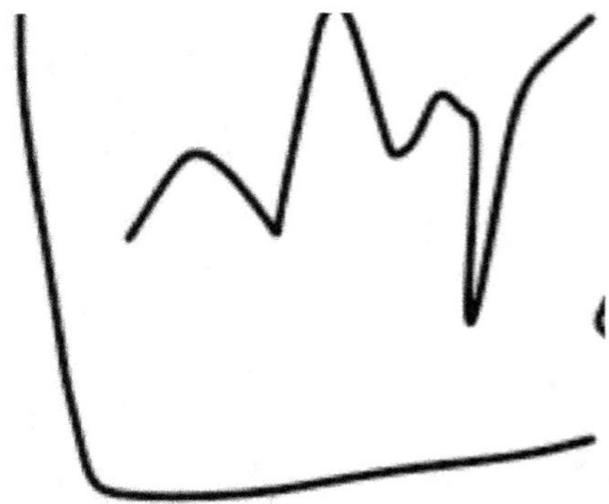

get. * *this is supposed to look like a data point, a graph*

Once you recognize the pattern, you can intervene anywhere. Flip the limiting paradigm to create a desired state.

Something interesting to note, is that when you focus on the thinking patterns that contribute to the state, or mood (emotion, feeling), and you recognize that when you care about yourself enough to shift your thinking to align with a desired, or preferred, way to feel (balanced - not too much, not too little, enough) it takes the focus off of behavior. Our behavior, what we do or don't do, will become a natural, or flowing, part of our experience as it is driven by an inspired, or balanced state.

If your belief in self-care is an action, a do, a behavior, it may not shift your feeling state. You can go get a pedicure, but if you have not shifted your thinking to create or allow a state of balance, then you are getting a pedicure as an observable action or behavior, but your inside world may not be demonstrating a state that is contributing to feeling good.

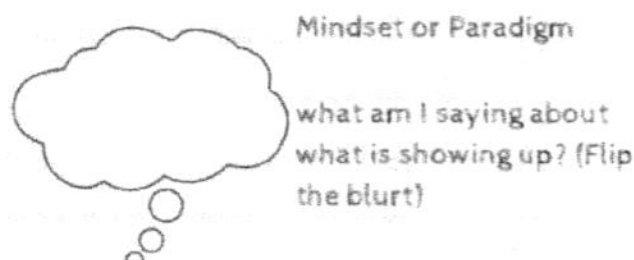

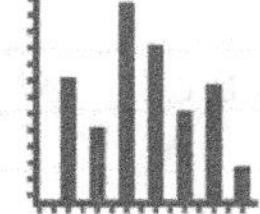

Actions/Non Actions

Observable - what am I doing or not doing? (our behavior can become more natural and 'easy' when we focus on thinking thoughts, or telling a story, that matches a desireable state: balance – not too much, not too little, enough.

see.feel.do.get.

The goal is to feel good. Our energetic state is vibrational. Just like we don't doubt, or argue, the law of gravity; we need not doubt, or argue, the theory of relativity. We attract at a vibrational level. Like energy creates like energy. Our thoughts create a feeling state. The energetic feeling state summons our interpretation of what we experience. We create the filter, we tell the story. The skill of self-awareness allows us to notice our thoughts. When we notice limiting thoughts, we can choose to disrupt the pattern and tell our own story. The story that allows for what IS possible. This story creates an energetic feeling state of possibility. Now we attract at this higher vibrational state. Anything can happen. Anything is possible. Now THIS is me.

Epilogue

Parts one, two, and three were originally pieces of online courses I began to create in January 2020. A friend of mine, who took the first course, self-care, suggested that I should have began the course with this conclusion. My life is transformed. All the skills, tools, and strategies I share are those that I use regularly, or have used but are no longer relevant. The following is the conclusion I wrote in January 2020.

While preparing to publish this first monthly course, I contemplated my own growth.

I haven't had a depressive episode in longer than I can remember. I can say with confidence that it has been at least two years, maybe even three.

Not only have I not had an episode, I haven't even felt the familiar tinge of 'warning' that I came to know so well. The sensation of the *Big Feeling*...the dark cloud looming over head, with the storm in the distance...that has taught me, over time, if I engage with it, I loop in to its cycle.

Overwhelm. Powerless. Longing. These feelings show up. I notice them. I name them. I choose to allow the feeling, knowing that by allowing I am releasing the momentum. And as I continue to practice notice.name.allow.release., the intensity lessens.

The feelings are not in charge any more. They may show up, and stay for a bit longer than I care for them to, but underneath the discomfort is a knowing they are passing.

Another nudge that showed up this morning was a reminder of two big 'aha's' that shifted my experience of what I call 'ordinary day'. The first aha was maybe a little less than five years ago. While in the process of learning, applying, and teaching skills, I realized that there were two people I was allowing a lot of power to trigger BIG emotional responses inside of me. To be clear, it wasn't the human person, as much as it was the belief I had about the role they represented in my life.

I realized that by giving them this power, I needed them to see me, to really hear me, to fully understand me, and to value my existence. I was spinning in a cycle of emotional unease because the two people I gave this power to, over and over again, were not seeing me for who I knew myself to be. Because they didn't 'see' me, then for sure they didn't 'hear' what I wanted them to hear, and of course if they didn't see or hear me as I desired, then how could they 'understand' and 'value' me.

It wasn't their job to.

When I finally came to this realization, I turned everything toward me. I did two things. I saw myself. I listened to myself with the intent to hear. I connected to, and understood, ME. I valued ME, and began to affirm ME. I then recognized that if I wanted the validation from them, then maybe there were others in my life who wanted, or would appreciate, this validation from me. I began to turn it around and practice seeing others for who they were, to listen with the intent to hear, to try to understand, and to value that they existed.

Shift.

The other big game changer was maybe three summers ago. I had a depressive episode show up. I was enraged. The hateful talk showed up and I finally recognized it, I caught it. I recognized that this was where it could change. I had gone months without an episode, I had made massive growth. It wasn't about the absence of the depression (depression wasn't an enemy), it was an understanding. I also learned that when the *Big Feelings* show up, it's an opportunity to let them go. To release the power. To comfort and soothe myself by the story I choose to tell. The power, or the momentum, lessens. Eventually there is space. Space to stay in charge. To control how I respond. To fully be aware and to fully choose the path I want to take, recognizing that engaging (in my case, it was abusive, hateful self-talk) was only going to create more of the same.

Can you see the self-care in the shifting, or healing, process? Caring about yourself. Caring about how you feel.

One last thing, I could go on and on about observable and practical, daily practices that have become part of my routine that fit into this 'self-care' lens. When I use the term self-care, I am referring to caring about yourself enough to begin a practice of self-awareness that brings you into your body to recognize sensations that are cueing you all the time as to what 'state' you are in. What story are you telling about the sensations? You get to tell your own story. The story shifts the state. Intuition and broad view live in the expansive state of wellbeing. Attune yourself to your own guidance. You'll get it. And when you do, you get to share it with others.

appendix

1. List 5 influential people, ideas, or things relevant to your life right now.

- yoga
- matt
- smoosh
- online course creation
- residual income

2. Now write at least one quality for each choice that really stands out.

calming and beautiful

powerful and vulnerable

pure love

creative, exciting, and fun

fun flowing

Who am I?

Introduce yourself using the qualities you listed...

Sally's presence is instantly calming.
Sally radiates pure love and is fun to be around.
Sally is powerful in the way her creative ideas are
constantly flowing,
yet there is a vulnerability that is beautiful.
It is exciting to be around Sally.

Ask yourself...

<u>example</u>:

What breaks my heart?

when someone is not heard - like they don't matter

What makes me feel most alive?

to feel inspired and to inspire others

Create a mission statement by declaring a statement that combines your greatest heartbreak and your greatest joy.

example

Sally creates and shares ideas that allow adults and children to feel seen, heard, valued and understood.

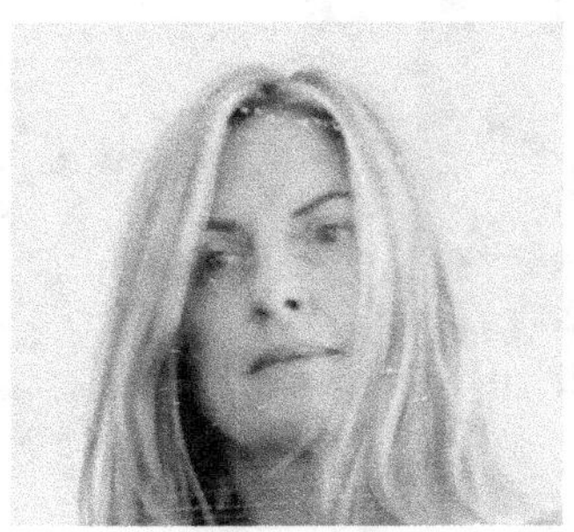

About the Author

I am a public academic working in schools since 1995.

In 2007, I received my MSW from the University of Denver and began working as a school social worker in the greater Denver area. I became passionate about mindfulness and teacher self-care as essential interventions in response to school violence and student death by suicide.

I define self-care as caring about yourself enough to notice your thoughts and the story they tell; then choosing skills, tools, and strategies to shift limiting scripts. I have over 25 years of experience with all grade levels across three states: Illinois, California, and Colorado.

Over the last ten years, I have created several curriculum concepts that include the *checkIN* and *Movement.Breath.Kindness.* In June 2020, I published the *storyitell* ebook: *The Story I Tell. How to make the Age of Disruption work for you.* In addition to the ebook, there is a companion eworkbook that makes it simple to transfer the skills, tools, and strategies to a classroom or coaching session. *Storyitell* is now available in paperback at Amazon.com. In January 2021 I published a second ebook: *Something More. Connecting to the pulse of a Shared Humanity.* January 2022 I published a third ebook: *abetterway. Using*

Inner Resources to Create Your Own Algorithm. All books are now available in paperback at Amazon books.

I publish a weekly blog at sallyseifferco.blog that is posted on Sally & Sifer Facebook Page. I publish weekly content on Instagram @sallysifer, as well as visual content that complements blog posts on the Sally & Sifer YouTube channel, TikTok, and Instagram Reels.

Summer 2022 began an 8-week teaching series that began June 4 on @sallysifer Facebook Page. Additionally, 2022 8-week teaching series can be found on the FB page beginning on January 24 and April 4. A recent 8-week series focused on *The Story I Tell* began on January 17, 2023 and ended March 13, 2023. Check out the *storyitell* blogs 1–8 for content.

You can connect with me on:
- https://sallyseifferco.blog
- https://www.facebook.com/sallysifer
- https://www.instagram.com/sallysifer
- https://www.youtube.com/sallysifer
- https://www.tiktok.com/@sallysifer